SEIZE THE DAY

One Girl's Inspirational Story of
Growing Up and Learning to Live
a Happy, Healthy Life with Epilepsy

~~~~~~

ABBY GUSTUS ALFORD

SEIZE THE DAY

One Girl's Inspirational Story of Growing Up and Learning to
Live a Happy, Healthy Life with Epilepsy

Front cover photograph by Katie Alexander Alford

www.SeizeTheDayAbby.com

FIRST EDITION

Published by Adriel Publishing
Printed in the U.S.A.
ISBN: 978-1-892324-32-0

To my fellow epileptics and the family and friends who love them.

And for my family and friends, for loving me always.

CONTENTS

Forward

Prologue

Chapter 1:   *Choose the Bright Side from the Start*

Chapter 2:   *Roots*

Chapter 3:   *The Declaration*

Chapter 4:   *The Next Step*

Chapter 5:   *In Pursuit of Answers*

Chapter 6:   *Knowledge is Power*

Chapter 7:   *Places to Go, People to Meet*

Chapter 8:   *A Mind of My Own*

Chapter 9:   *Big Cities, Bigger Dreams*

Chapter 11:   *Right Where I Need to Be*

Chapter 12:   *Reflections*

FORWARD

~~~~~~~~~~

By Christine Gustus

"Abby's declared herself. She has a seizure disorder." Those words, uttered by the doctor, will forever stay with me. I was devastated. Our precious daughter was diagnosed with epilepsy, and we were about to begin a journey that our family had not bargained for.

There were countless doctor visits, tons of medical tests, and all different medications used to treat Abby, but nothing seemed to help during those first tumultuous weeks and months after her diagnosis. I felt like our life had been turned upside down.

We had a beautiful, successful teenage daughter who was angry and resentful that she had to deal with epilepsy. As I look back she fought taking her medication and visits to the doctor every step of the way. It was a daily challenge for our family to protect her and keep her safe.

I wanted Abby to take her medicine on a regular basis— every twelve hours. I bought every type of pill box, so she would keep the tablets of medicine with her at all times. She would leave the house for a weekend activity, and I would find the pill box stashed in her room or the bathroom. She would then suffer another seizure because she missed a dose of medicine. How would we ever help her if she did not cooperate and follow the doctor's instructions?

Getting Abby through high school was a very difficult time for us. She had break through seizures at night when she was sleeping. I clearly remember one night when we heard Abby fall out of bed. Her dad and I ran into her room, only to find her on the floor in a full-blown seizure. Her eyes rolled back in her head, she was rigid, her teeth were clamped together, and she was shaking uncontrollably. After the seizure was over, we got her back into bed so she could sleep and recover. When we got back in bed, I looked over at my husband and he had tears running down his face. He did not want to talk about it, so we went back to sleep feeling sadness and grief. That was moment I realized that the seizures were affecting both of us.

The seizure disorder affected my husband and me, yes, but it affected her brother, Byron, as well. I recall the day that he had a disagreement with me. He said to me, "You are always helping Abby, but you ignore me." It was at that moment I realized we were making accommodations for Abby and her epilepsy, but not attending to the needs of her brother. I apologized to him and made a concerted effort to care for his wants and needs as much as I cared for Abby's.

Another memorable incident occurred while we were at dinner with my extended family—my sisters and nephews. We were at a local restaurant having dinner. Abby was getting her hamburger just the way she wanted it and looked at the ketchup and said, "Please pass the red." I looked at her terrified and wondered if the seizures were causing word-finding problems. Had we entered another stage in our journey with epilepsy? I knew we needed to find another doctor to see if he could help her.

We did locate a wonderful doctor at Children's Hospital in St. Louis, and we believed we had found someone who would help us. Even though Abby was resistant and not sure if she liked this particular doctor, her father and I did.

This wonderful pediatric neurologist prescribed medicine that did not have as many side effects. She was getting ready to leave for college, so we knew that we needed a better combination of medicines so she would be able to function in her new environment.

She chose to attend Purdue University to my delight since that was my alma mater. Luckily for her father and me, she ended up with a roommate, Kelley, who we saw as an angel from heaven. She seemed to be there whenever Abby's seizures occurred and always provided her the love and care she needed.

One day when Abby was out of college and in the workplace, I finally saw a more grown up version of our daughter. We were sitting in the living room and she said, "I don't want to have these seizures anymore. I can't remember so many events from my past. What do I need to do?" I felt at that moment we crossed an important barrier she had had up for so many years.

I replied that it is important to take her medicine regularly, eat a healthy diet, and get enough sleep. Those were a few modifications she could make to her lifestyle that would help to change the outcome of her seizure disorder. To my delight she took the advice and began working on her own health, and we saw a significant decrease in her seizures.

There are some long-lasting effects of epilepsy we see today. Abby's memory of special events or times from high school is gone. I might say, "Remember when we…." and Abby responds in the negative. She, to this day, has no recollection of the events we often discuss as a family. The seizures have erased them from her memory. It makes me sad that she cannot recall special times.

Abby will share with you the recollections she has from her journey with epilepsy and the bond we have with her. I'm proud to say, we remained close during all of the time we were trying to navigate this difficult seizure disorder.

I am happy to tell you that Abby has done well, and we remain a close knit family. *Seize the Day* will give insight to her journey and hope for families finding their way through the many trials and tribulations of the epilepsy journey.

The First Night of the Rest of My Life

"We must be willing to let go of the life we planned,

so as to have the life that is waiting for us."

JOSEPH CAMPBELL

The first time it happened, I was 12 years old. I was at an out-of-town softball tournament with my mom and little brother, Byron. I played on an elite team that traveled almost every weekend, which got expensive so we stayed in the cheaper hotels when we could, and the one we were in that night was pretty dingy.

The look of the room is etched in my memory forever. There were two beds. Each bed had a navy comforter with ugly pink and maroon flowers –– the kind you could find in an old worn down house with outdated décor (or your grandmother's house if your grandma is anything like mine). The carpet was a deep red. I remember distinctly that it did not match the bed and it's worn out comforter. There was a small wooden table with two chairs at the very back of the room and a small black tube TV placed on a wooden dresser directly in front of both beds in the middle. There was a nightstand in between the two beds. Of course, it was wood also, but one that didn't match the other two.

I find it funny that I remember this night so distinctly. I never, ever (after this first seizure) could remember anything like this again… unless I really thought about it, made an effort and told myself… remember this.

It never takes me long to fall asleep, and this night was no different. In fact, I pretty much just hit the pillow and was out. I was in the bed closest to the door with my little brother Byron. I'm pretty sure he fell asleep as fast as I did, but it wasn't long before I would wake him up.

Then, it happened. My arms started flailing around, and my body became rigid. Byron was convinced I was hitting him and just playing around.

We had a game growing up where we would give each other a hard punch in the arm or leg (some people call it a "charlie horse") and yell "CORKER." My dad came up with it as a joke. So, Byron automatically assumed this was a game. He has told me many times since that night that is what he was convinced was happening. He, of course, thinking I was playing around proceeded to hit me back and yell, "CORKER."

It became clear quickly that this was not a game and I was not playing around. If only that was the case. Something else was going on.

My head was violently arched back to my right. My body was stiff as a board. My eyes rolled back in my head, and I was blinking uncontrollably. I was unconscious. I was having my very first grand mal seizure.

While I was unconscious during the actual seizure, throughout the night I would come in and out of consciousness. I have very distinct and accurate memories of what happened. My mom, Byron and I have all talked about it on numerous occasions, and they are amazed at the accuracy of my recollection. We've talked about it a lot, because this was a night that changed all of our lives, not just mine.

My mom flipped on the light on the nightstand in between our two beds after Byron started screaming. A moment of shock set in for Byron and he started crying. Byron and my mom had no idea what was going on. I was shaking uncontrollably... not just uncontrollably, I was shaking violently. I also started foaming at the mouth. When they both called my name, there was no response.

"Abby," my mom screamed.

"What's going on? Abby!!!" Byron yelled.

My mom was panicking. In the midst of the chaos, my mom called 911.

I know my mom had no idea, at this point, what was really going on. Neither did Byron. After what seemed like an eternity, but was only about two full minutes, I stopped the violent movements and my body slowly relaxed. My dad always says, "Even when you know what's happening and know it will end, it still seems like the longest two or three minutes of your life."

I was lying there like a limp dog, or more accurately, a dead dog. I had no control of any of my limbs. I couldn't speak. I'm not really sure what all my brother and my mom tried to get me to do or say as they waited for the paramedics.

My mom said after the fact, when I was old enough to start understanding how hard this was on the people around me, "Here is my beautiful, talented daughter... my daughter who has the world at her fingertips and she can't walk, she can't talk, she can't

13

do anything. It was awful, Abby, just awful."

Still today, she can tell that story and inevitably her eyes will well up with tears, as do mine. I hear what she went through that night, the fear she and Byron felt and want to cry myself. Those 30 minutes to an hour where you are conscious, but cannot talk or walk or really comprehend what is going on around you, is known as the postictal phase. It's a critical phase of having a seizure that people unfamiliar with epilepsy need to know about. It's a short period of time after grand mal seizures and people are completely unresponsive.

My mom always says the instant I could not talk or walk or even stand up she thought her life had changed forever… well, it had. I just think to myself now that it was not necessarily as bad as maybe she had originally thought. Now that period of time doesn't terrify her half as badly as it did that night. She understands my postictal phase and what to expect.

The next time I regained consciousness I was actually sitting up on the side of the bed… a very good sign by any stretch. A male paramedic, with short blond-hair (I have no other details for you, but I remember he was good-looking, which makes the state I was in even more embarrassing), was kneeling right in front of me. He had one hand on my chin holding my head up, and he was asking me questions.

I'm pretty sure I couldn't answer them, or at least I have no recollection of answering any of the simple questions I was being asked. He was probably asking me questions like, what is your name? Where are you from? How old are you? Those are questions I know I am not able to answer right after I have a seizure.

As he was holding up my head, I remember looking at him

with a blank stare during the questioning period and getting very scared about not knowing the answers. I looked up from his gaze and saw my mom.

I have seen my mom upset, I have seen her sick. She has terrible migraines, so I have seen her at her worst. Nothing could ever compare to how distraught she was when I looked up at her. She was standing behind the paramedic. Another paramedic was standing next to her looking like she was trying to comfort her. She was sobbing. Her face was bright red. She had one hand crossed across her body and the other was up with her hand across her mouth. She was still in her light blue nightgown.

I looked up at her as tears were streaming down her face and said in one single breath, "MOM???"

I didn't get out, "What is going on?" She must have known that is what I meant from my eyes. I was crying too, scared to death about what was going on even though my moment of consciousness was so incredibly brief.

She shook her head, shrugged her shoulders as she cried even harder, swaying back and forth in a frantic and said, "I don't know, Ab, I don't know."

And... I blacked out again.

It's terribly difficult to explain her hysterical state, but seeing her that terrified and upset made me scared to death about what was happening.

Soon after, they brought in the gurney. I'm assuming they had to lift me on, as I could still do nothing for myself.

Randomly, once again, I woke up. This time I was being rolled through the middle of the hallway. I had an IV in my arm, and an oxygen mask covering my face so I couldn't talk. The paramedic, was once again, standing above me pushing the gurney and the other paramedic who was originally standing next to my mom was at the foot of the gurney wheeling it along.

When I woke up this time, I didn't see Byron or my mom. This scared me, but I was so fatigued, I could not have gotten a word out if I had tried. I remember waking up, seeing these things around me, feeling dizzy, thinking oh my god, my body feels exhausted and weak. I had no other option but to fall right back asleep. I saw all of those things around me, but did not have the capacity to really absorb, comprehend or respond to what was going on.

THE NEXT DAY

I have no idea what time it was the next day when I woke up. I 'came to' in a hospital room. When you have epilepsy and you say that you 'came to,' it simply means you are now aware of your surroundings and no longer unconscious or in the postictal phase.

I woke up in a bed with a mint colored-curtain pulled around the room and it looked like more of an Emergency Room-type room than a hospital room where you would actually be admitted. My mom and my mom's friend, Mickey, were standing next to the bed. Mickey was a family friend of ours. Her daughter, Jenny, was on my softball team, and her husband happened to be our coach. They were very close family friends at the time so it was only natural she was there with us.

I was dazed and in a hazy fog, although, I could finally comprehend what was going on around me. My body felt like it had been hit by a truck, but laying there in that bed, I was not fully aware of how bad I felt. I looked up and smiled when I turned my head and saw my mom. She gave me a half smile back.

I think she was still completely terrified by the situation that was unfolding. I can honestly say that I did not care. I only had one thought. When can I get back to my softball tournament? I wanted to be on the field as soon as possible. Looking back now, it's surprising to me that I only wanted to know when I could get back to my tournament. But, I was only 12, and in a 12 year old's mind, sports and friends are about the only things that matter, at least that is how it was for me.

I did not care why I was in the hospital. I did not care about what happened the night before. I did not care what the doctors and nurses said every time they came in the room. I sure as hell had no interest in all of the questions they asked me and tests they wanted to run on me. It went something like medical history questions, blood work, CT Scan, MRI, more medical history questions, more blood work, and more basic questions to see if I knew my name, where I lived, and my birthday.

All of it did not matter. In my head I felt "okay enough" to get up and go. But, that was the problem, it was in my head. I had no idea how tired my body was. I wanted to play.

Softball tournaments were all day Saturday and Sunday. If you were coming up through the losers bracket on Sunday, your team could easily play five or six games in one day. That was the case for my team that Sunday. My seizure happened Saturday night, which only meant, we were coming up from the losers bracket and if we did not lose, we were playing for the championship later that day. In my head, it was single elimination, single elimination, single elimination. Every game mattered. Again, at 12 years old, I had blinders on. At the time, the seriousness of the situation meant nothing to me. Being in the hospital was just a nuisance... a complete waste of my time.

"When can I go back and play?"

"You're not going to play this weekend, Ab."

I looked at Mrs. Cervetto as if she had the power to override this decision. After all, her husband was the coach.

"Yeah, honey, you can't play for the rest of the weekend, until we figure out what's going on."

"What?!?!" I felt tired and weak, but I was strong willed and not about to let someone tell me I couldn't do something. "NO!" I said. I was determined to get on the field.

I started crying again, "I have to play! I want to play, get me out of here! Please, Mom, please! Don't do this to me!"

It was true, I was way too weak to play the day after my very first grand mal seizure. But, while I was just lying in that hard, uncomfortable bed my body felt fine. I could talk again, I could walk again (I thought), I knew where I was and why I was there. I truly believed I was okay and ready to get back on the field.

After being told no, I was crying again. I was not sobbing, I just had tears running down my face. I rolled my eyes and looked away from them and stared at that ugly hospital curtain. The last time I cried I was in the hotel room and terrified. This time, I was not scared. I would have walked away mad, but I had a few IVs in my arm and was still really tired... and so I just laid there. I laid there bored and frustrated. I had nothing to say to my mom or Mrs. Cervetto. Now, I was just mad. No, I was pissed. Pissed at the world, and even more so, pissed at my mom and pissed at the situation.

The doctors confirmed it was a grand mal seizure that day. In my eyes, it was a good thing they could tell us what happened and also about damn time… they only ran 8,000 tests. Still, though, we had no idea why it happened.

I slept in the hospital pretty much non-stop except for a few small interactions with the doctors and nurses and that one small interaction with my mom and Mrs. Cervetto. My body was way more tired than my head would allow me to think it was. My body would have failed me that day, I just did not know it.

I still, to this day, want to believe that I could have rallied. My adult self knows better. I know now that it would not be a good idea to get up. Any kind of physical activity at that point would be out of the question, I just did not know that yet. My adult self knows I need to stay in bed for a day after a seizure.

Ultimately, my mom, Mrs. Cervetto, and the doctors who kept me there nearly all day were right. I might have lasted ten minutes on the field, probably not even that long.

Up until that night of my life, I had never had any real health issues.

I had never broken a bone. I hardly ever got sick. I sure as hell had never been hospitalized. I was a healthy 12 year old!

What in the world was going on? Was this seizure a fluke? Was my life changed forever?

The answer was simple, but I didn't know it yet. This was not a fluke and yes. Yes, your life is changed forever.

Abby's Advice

Abby's Advice is a column with information and little tidbits that I wish my loved ones and I had known when we began this epilepsy journey. It may come in the form of questions to ask or consider for your next doctor appointment or just a small piece of advice and encouragement to have in your back pocket. They'll be popping up throughout this book and are designed to be short and sweet take-aways. I encourage you to really embrace the advice and write it down... plug it in to your phone if it resonates with you or post it on social media, or if you're really wild and crazy... tattoo it on your forehead! Just kidding... But seriously, use this advice to your advantage. And now, our first *Abby's Advice*...

Abby's Advice

When you see a person have a seizure, call 911 if...

- The person has never had a seizure before
- The person can't wake up after the seizure
- The seizures lasts more than three minutes
- The person has multiple seizures in a row
- The person is physically hurt
- The seizure happens in water
- The person has another health condition that may cause additional problems

ONE

Choose the Bright Side from the Start

"Life is 10% of what happens to you and 90% how you react to it."

CHARLES R. SWINDOLL

My first seizure was traumatic. I'm not going to lie. Every seizure always is, but there's something to be said for that initial terror that rocks an entire family to its core. I have so many different stories, different experiences, and different emotions with epilepsy, that I will get to later in the book, but it's important for me that my readers get to know me as a person. Before you start to hear and relate to the terrible traumas of epilepsy, I want to show you who I am as a person. I want to help you get to know me, and what has over time, made me, well... me.

So, let's dive right in and start with the title of this book. I know the word "seize" in the epilepsy community can be a bit controversial. In fact, there have been negative articles written about people who have said it... but why?!? Seizing is bad, yes. I get that. But when people say "Seize the Day," it's a good thing. Nobody is saying that in reference to somebody having a seizure...

they just aren't. And, neither am I!

All my life I grew up saying "Seize the Day" and it was always a really good thing. It was never a bad thing… why should it be now? It's a positive saying and one that all people, yes, even people outside our epilepsy community, understand. And, that's where we (as a community) need to focus our attention. We need that help, help to bring awareness and help to raise money for research. Let's not only accept this but fully embrace it!

I am here to share my traumatic stories, but through those, I also hope to inspire families across the world just like mine. I want all people to know a happy and healthy life is 100 percent possible. Epilepsy is a part of me, and yes, it's a definitive part of me that has shaped who I am today. But, overcoming all of those hardships, that's what has made me the successful and happy adult that I am today. I never had it easy, and much of that is because of this disorder, but that is okay. It makes me unique, it makes me special, and it makes me Abby.

No doubt about it, the stories you'll read can be sad and disheartening. Whether it is you having the seizures, or somebody you love, the language of emotions felt is universal. Everyone can relate to those emotions.

There's no doubt, my naturally positive outlook was tested, but the people who loved me forced me to focus on the good in life. That shaped my attitude and made me always look at situations and say, "yes, but, on the bright side…". And, that's where I choose to stay, even now, on the bright side. And, whenever opportunities come my way, once again, the people around me have always wanted me to, yes, "seize" them! So here I am today, living my life on "the bright side" ready to "seize the day."

This outlook, in my opinion, speaks to how I was raised and my family, friends, and medical professionals along the way who loved me unconditionally.

Please note, I've changed the names of the doctors in the book to protect their identities. I believe all of my doctors have helped me tremendously, but I wanted to be respectful of their privacy. As a family, we love golf. That said, in this book, the doctors who treated me are named after two of our favorite golfers.

Now... back to my journey.

BACK TO REALITY

Going back to school on the Monday morning after my very first seizure was a whirlwind. By that time, I had for the most part fully recovered from my seizure. I was still slightly traumatized by the weekend, but nothing was wrong physically, and my strength was back. But, things had changed. My mom had to come with me to school that morning and explain to all my teachers that I had a seizure that weekend. Some people did not even know what a seizure was. I'm not going to lie, up until that point in my life, I didn't either.

My mom had to explain to all the school administrators that we had no idea if me having this grand mal seizure was a complete fluke or if I would have another one that day in front of all my friends and teachers. It was a possibility. I was taking medicine, but there are no cures for seizures. It's not guaranteed to be controlled when you take medicine. It's not an illness, where you can go home, take an antibiotic, and be fine in 24 hours.

In addition to that, there is no way to determine when a

seizure might happen. Some people with seizures can feel one coming on, but I was asleep when it first happened so at this point in time, I had no clue what to expect if a seizure was about to happen.

I'll never forget the fear I felt standing in the hall that morning. I was in sixth grade, and the fact that Abby Gustus had a seizure over the weekend was *huge* news. A couple of my close friends found out, because they saw my mom at school, and of course, that is not normal. So, I told them what happened.

For the most part, I was a confident sixth grader. I had tons of friends and was pretty happy go lucky. That day, I remember wanting to hide in my half size super small upper locker. Anywhere in the world would have been better than standing in that sixth grade hallway. It felt like person after person was coming up to me and asking me questions. I knew what happened over the weekend, but didn't know how to describe it to anybody at that point.

And, at that point, my diagnosis was not epilepsy. It was only one seizure. One event of abnormal electrical activity – too many neurons firing messages at one time in my brain. I had one grand mal seizure, otherwise known as a generalized tonic-clonic seizure, and that was it. We did not know why. We did not know if it would happen again. We knew, well, basically nothing.

As more and more people came up to me, "Abby, did you really have a seizure this weekend?" I would embarrassingly half smile and say yes, simultaneously wishing the locker was bigger so I could get in it. I stood there and answered the questions as well as I could until the bell rang. Thank god for the first period bell. And, even more importantly, thank god we were in sixth grade.

By lunch, there was something else to talk about.

MY FIRST DOCTOR'S VISIT

That whole week, my mom and dad were in full blown "find-the-best-doctor-in-the-world" mode. I had to get in to the doctor fast, because I needed a prescription for anti-seizure medication.

I'm not going to lie. My parents did all of this research for me. I did not schedule the appointments. I did not research the doctors. I did not pick the doctor we saw. I was 12 and let my parents handle it. Either way, I know now, that the doctor I saw the week after I had my first seizure was one of the very best pediatric neurologists in St. Louis. His name was Dr. Nicklaus.

I remember walking into his office later that week. It was all dark wood, like the color of mahogany, with built in book shelves that went all the way to the ceiling. He had a huge desk in front of his built-in book shelves with two visitor chairs sitting there, inviting my mom and me to take a seat. His office reminded me more of a college professor's office than a doctor's office. The amount of books he had was incredible. I remember thinking about it, because I love books.

We all shook hands, briefly introduced ourselves, and took a seat.

It's interesting when you are a child. The doctors (at least all of mine) always look straight at my mom or dad, whoever happens to be there, and ask them the standard questions. They would never look at me and say, "Abby, what happened? Tell me what's going on."

I understand that it is sometimes easier to talk directly to the parents about epilepsy and what actually happened during the seizure, but it would be awesome if somebody would have just asked me.

Either way, I wasn't planning on this being a long term relationship, so I just let it be. The visit, in my opinion, was extremely short. My mom answered all the questions Dr. Nicklaus asked. She explained what happened that night. She explained the violent grand mal seizure I had in the hotel room in bed while lying next to my brother.

She explained how we spent the next 24 hours after the seizure running every test imaginable in the Emergency Room. She explained all the results, which of course, showed no root cause.

I stayed quiet and listened while thinking in my head this would be my first and last "visit" with Dr. Nicklaus. Ultimately, we walked out of the doctor optimistic that this seizure was a fluke. This type of thing happens to a lot of kids. This would probably never happen again.

Dr. Nicklaus prescribed Depakote, an anti-convulsant medication, with the intention of slowly weening me off of it within two months.

Two months came and went before I knew it. I was on Depakote and turned into a zombie. This seizure medication changed my life, and not for the better. Did I have a seizure while I was taking the medication? No. Did I have any sort of quality of life? No. I slept all the time. It was hard to stay awake at school. I felt like I always wanted my bed. My eyelids were heavy and focusing on tasks at school was nearly impossible. This could not be normal.

To this day, I cringe (and get a little angry) when I talk to a person with epilepsy that has been prescribed Depakote. It makes me mad that in the 21st Century, this is what the medical community would consider a solution to seizures. Let me just say for the record, the Gustus family was not accepting this as a solution. This drug was not going to work for me or for the people who loved me.

Back then our thought process was different. Soon enough, I'd be off of it, so did it really matter? Before we knew it, I'd be taking less and less each week, so did it really matter? In our minds, at that point in time, the answer was no. My mom, dad, and I all believed that this was a fluke, and as soon as I was off the medicine, that terrible night would be a distant memory.

It's no surprise that my energy levels started slowly getting better the less Depakote I took. I was becoming my normal self again. I felt fantastic! I took my last dose and felt like throwing a party. No more medicine! It was euphoria. It's kind of amazing that one small pill can alter your entire life.

Abby's Advice

Always ask the doctors about medication side effects before accepting a prescription. If it's your first visit, ask how long the drug has been on the market to treat epilepsy. Chances are... if it's greater than 20 years old, there's something else out there that is worth asking about. If the doctor prescribes an older medication, accept it, but ask about the newer ones. Write down the name and research it later. Then, come prepared for your next visit.

To receive your FREE **Top 5 Tips for Parents and Teens** *go to www.SeizeTheDayAbby.com and enter your name and E-mail.*

TWO

Roots

~~~~~~~~~~~~~~~~~~~~~~~~~~~~~~~~~~~

"Family is not an important thing, it's everything."

MICHAEL J. FOX

After I got off the anti-seizure medication, my life returned to normal… not just for me, but for my entire family… and yes, that even included my extended family. My grandparents were heavily involved in everything we did growing up, and I'm sure many of you can relate when I say, seizures affect families, not just individuals. That said, let me tell you a little bit about them.

WHERE IT ALL BEGAN

My dad, Doyle, grew up all across the United States because my grandpa worked on the railroad and moved often to manage different job sites. He spent all of his summers with his best friend and cousin, Kem, in a small town called Fort Gibson, Okla. which is where his mother, my grandma, is from. It's one of my very favorite places to visit, and I'm proud to have family from small town America. My grandma's name is Opal and she had three sisters, Diamond, Ruby, and Pearl. That is always my fun fact about myself any time I have to play an icebreaker game for a team building activity no matter where it may be. Nobody can ever guess it's me, considering I grew up in St. Louis, and most people I meet already know that fun fact due to my outspoken love of the St. Louis Cardinals and Blues.

My dad's family in Fort Gibson all lived on the same farm. As we've gotten older, it's gotten smaller, but it's definitely a very close group.

I got to go to Fort Gibson on occasion growing up. My cousins would take me back-roading and taught us about what it was like to grow up on a farm. It was definitely different from what I was used to in St. Louis, but I appreciated the fact that it was part of my dad's background.

My dad is an only child and moved to St. Louis once he was a teenager after criss-crossing the U.S. with his dad and mom, who I call Pop-pop and Granny, most of his childhood. My paternal grandparents were fantastic people. They both retired early, so I spent all of my sick days, snow days, pretty much any day we had off school, with them, because both of my parents worked. My brother and I spent our summers at the country club close to their house playing golf and swimming. Pop-pop would golf with Byron and me when we weren't at the pool.

Pop-pop was the grandpa who picked us up from school and drove us to piano lessons. All of my classmates also knew my Pop-pop, because he was a staple figure at activities and picked us up so often. He taught me to drive and took me to get my driver's license the day I turned 16.

His favorite thing to say to me was, "You're my favorite granddaughter."

I would laugh at him, and say, "I'm your *only* granddaughter."

He would say, "Yes, but your still my favorite."

I still think about that and smile. I miss him... a lot.

Granny loved my brother and me just as much. Ruby would always tell me, "You know you are the light of your Granny's life, right? She loves you and is so proud of you and Byron."

There was never a doubt about that, we always knew.

My mom grew up in St. Louis. We called my mom's mom and dad, Grandma Fran and Buddy. My grandpa was a very successful business man. He had his hands in many different businesses my whole life. He had an entrepreneurial spirit and passed along amazing business advice to me all through my early 20s.

My Grandma Fran was the woman I always want to be just like. She was the classiest, kind-hearted lady I've ever met in my life. She had perfectly manicured nails and perfect hair and make-up always. She was beautiful inside and out. Growing up, I played dress up in her closet, and she let me take a new Chanel lipstick home with me every time I went over there. To this day, I only buy Chanel lipstick. It's a habit.

I was the only granddaughter on that side of the family until I was a teenager, so it's safe to say, I was a little bit spoiled when holidays rolled around. Grandma Fran always made sure I was dressed to the nines. All. The. Time. Every Saturday growing up, my mom, Grandma Fran, and I would "do lunch and shop."

Our favorite stops were Nordstrom and Talbots. I had cable knit cardigans in every color of the rainbow thanks to Grandma

Fran (and Buddy).

My mom was the second of four daughters. My aunts are named Anne, Joan, and Nancy. I am lucky enough to be extremely close to all of them. They all have been at every major event in my life. When I spoke at my high school graduation, they all made the trip to be there and see me. Anne and Nancy both live in California, and Joan and her family lived down the street from us in St. Louis. I consider Joan's kids, Ben, Danny, and Sam to be my brothers since we were always together growing up.

Buddy was very focused on our education. He made sure we all knew (all my cousins and me) that education was the most important thing in life. He would pay us $50 each summer to read six books and write book reports on them. Each grandkid had the same opportunity. If only somebody would pay me to read now, I'd be a rich woman! Back then, I was focused on playing outside and enjoying my summers. Now, though, I am 100 percent certain that my genuine love of reading comes from him. If you have any good book suggestions, please, send them my way!

Buddy also let me intern for a summer for his companies. He owned two at the time, and I asked him if I could help him in his "marketing department to get some experience." The department was non-existent, so I'm not sure what I was thinking, but I spent the summer by his side, learning about what he did and how he managed people and his companies. It taught me invaluable lessons about management, integrity, patience, and it was my introduction on how to run your own business. I was lucky to work for Buddy that summer and will always be grateful to him for that opportunity.

AS FOR THE REST...

My mom and dad are the definition of the All-American storybook tale. My dad was the football player, and my mom was the cheerleader. They dated all through high school and college. They parted ways for college. My dad had a football scholarship to Central Methodist University, and my mom headed off to Purdue University in West Lafayette, Ind. to get her Speech Pathology degree.

They ultimately both ended up back in St. Louis and got married shortly after. My mom and dad's love for each other, is the type of love I always wanted to find when I got married. Luckily, I did. My favorite thing about my parents is that they call each other "Ace." We always ask them how that started, and they just look at each other and laugh and say they have no idea! Either way, I think it speaks to their love and respect of one another.

My mom was a teacher, still is. She works with deaf kids and teaches them to talk. She is also a professor at Washington University in St. Louis. My mom is the type of lady who loves school. Most recently, she decided to go back to school at Lindenwood in St. Louis to get her Ed.D. in Instructional Leadership. She's 65! She's the eternal lover of learning. I can't blame her, I'm the same way. If I'm not doing something constantly to better myself, I'm always feeling a little bored. As we speak, I'm studying to get my real estate license. So, the apple does not fall far from the tree.

My mom is understanding, empathetic, encouraging, supportive, and kind. She has the best advice when it's needed, but the best ear when all you need is to talk it out. She is sensible enough to know the right time for that every time… which always helps. She never just gives advice for the sake of it, her advice is thoughtful and meaningful, and therefore I've always taken it to heart.

She has a great sense of humor, and when she laughs at a joke, her laugh is contagious and makes me laugh harder. That makes our relationship fun on top of everything else.

She's super positive, and it is infectious. Byron and I never needed an alarm clock. Every morning, my mom would open our doors and sing softly, *"Good Mornin'"* from *Singing in the Rain*, one of our all-time favorite movies.

"Good mornin', good mornin'
It's great to stay up late!
Good morning', good mornin'
To you!"

How's that for a wakeup call?! I know that sounds cheesy, but it's true. That is literally how I woke up every day my entire childhood. Byron too! I'm such a nerd, I made that song my alarm when I lived alone for the first time! That's a little embarrassing, but oh well… that song makes me happy.

Many of the children my mom works with have more problems than just being deaf. Before I had epilepsy, I was around children with disabilities all the time. The school for the deaf that my mom worked at was a boarding school. Many times, on holiday weekends, if the children's parents could not afford to fly them home, they would come to our house. She, and that meant we, welcomed them with open arms.

My mom would always say, "Nobody should ever be

alone at Christmas! If somebody is, we're having them over to our house!" That was how it was. She was inclusive and accepting of everyone. She taught me to be the same way, and that's something I'm proud of.

Having a disability was a hurdle, but that was all. My mom never treated the kids that would come to our house like they had a disability, and therefore, neither did we. Once I was diagnosed, I think my mom had the same mentality. She was never going to let me live my life differently. High expectations were maintained, and nothing changed.

I have tons of favorite stories about my mom, but one just makes me so happy when I think about it. I woke up one day in high school, and I just wasn't feeling that good. Could I have gone to school if I rallied? Yes. Did I want to go to school? No.

She came in my room to wake me up singing *"Good mornin'"* and looked at me.

"Mom, I don't feel very good."

"What's wrong?"

"I'm not really sure, I just don't feel great, and honestly, I want a little more time to study for that test."

She encouraged me to get up and go and told me I'd studied plenty and would do great on my test.

"But, I just feel bad."

"Okay," she said as she sat down on the side of the bed next to me. "You have to have these damn things, let's just take a day."

My face lit up! She meant since I've had to deal with all the B.S. that comes along with epilepsy, just this once, she was going to let me use it to my advantage! I was in high school, then, so first, I couldn't believe she said the word, damn, and second, that was cool. She didn't want me to ever be treated differently, but I realized that day that she knew I was slightly different. I also knew at that point, she thought seizures sucked really bad, too.

It meant the world to me that she let me stay home that day, not so much because I got out of going to school, but because I realized at that moment, my mom thought that it was unfair I had to deal with this, too.

That day I also knew my dad understood. Before he left that day, he knocked on the door and said, "feel better" and winked at me.

A weight was lifted off me that day. My parents and I were on the same page. Seizures sucked, damn it!

My dad was a stock broker and financial advisor. Today, he is a money manager and works for himself, just like Buddy always did.

My dad is hilarious, reliable, loving, smart, and a little on the strict side. Okay, a lot on the strict side. As a kid growing up, I thought my dad was super cool. I grew up, as I mentioned, with all boys, so I was a pretty big tomboy. We grew up going to the Lake of the Ozarks on the weekends. We fished, tubed, and water skied. He taught me to do all of it. I loved being on the water, and still to this day, water makes me feel happy and calm.

I think there is something about a childhood memory that can make you nostalgic. Being near boats and water does that for me, because it was such a major part of our lives, thanks to my dad.

He was a great teacher when it came to golf, softball, and soccer. He would pick me up when I was down and would be proud of me when I did well.

I know he was very proud of me when I made the Varsity

softball team as a freshman in the fall and then made the Varsity soccer team as a freshman in the spring. That was a big deal at the time. Lettering in two sports as a freshman was cool! I was proud, too.

High school was tough on our relationship, because I did not like to follow rules. He had tons of them, and I thought they were all stupid. We were both stubborn and not willing to budge, so that made it difficult. My mom was the peacekeeper in what she referred to as World War III.

The hardest rule for me to follow was curfew. I did not like having a midnight curfew when all my friends didn't have a curfew at all. I felt like it wasn't fair, but that was a rule set in stone for my parents. Needless to say, I was late… a lot. And, I was in trouble. Every. Single. Time. Now, staying up until midnight is nearly impossible. My how times have changed!

Today, I'm really glad I had *all* those rules, because it was apparent I needed them. I also know now, he was protecting me… protecting me from all things bad and I sincerely appreciate it as an adult. We were back to the relationship that I loved and cherished once I went to college.

My dad and I have a lighthearted, entertaining relationship. When I call (even now as an adult), he answers, "What do you want?" and it makes me laugh every single time… still after all these years! And, seriously, how did he know I wanted something!?! I'm just kidding (sort of).

As my career has slowly become more and more successful, he has become a confidant and mentor. As I navigate through corporate America, his advice is invaluable. For every situation that comes up, he's usually been there, done that. Then, he can steer me in the right direction.

One little piece of advice he gave me that is by far my favorite, "Believe me, in business, everything works out, it just always takes longer than you would like it to."

He gave me that advice when I was working for a really difficult boss. Turned out, he was right. Everything did work out, and just like he said, it was not on the timeline I wanted it to be, but things worked out. I always remind myself of that at work even today if I ever find myself doubting corporate decisions.

I love him for that among eight million other things.

My mom and dad tried for six years to have children before I was born. So, by the time I came around, I'm pretty sure they were very ready.

My piano teacher, who was very close to my parents, one time told me something that I will never forget, "You were a very wanted child, Abby, a blessing." That was something that stuck with me, and both my mom and my dad always treated Byron and me as blessings.

I had a very happy childhood. We grew up in a suburb of St. Louis called Chesterfield in a mid-size two story house on Appalachian Trail that was more than just a house, it was a home filled with love. My parents wanted Byron and me to be successful and gave us every opportunity to do so.

We were expected to do well in school. I remember one time getting knocked by my teacher for not knowing my basic multiplication tables in elementary school. Somehow I had faked that I knew them up to that point, but it caught up to me. My mom stayed up with me all night until I knew them all.

Byron and I were only a year and a half apart… two years

by grade in school. We were two peas in a pod. He was the classic younger brother. I teased him. I dared him to do crazy things and he did. I played pranks on him, and despite all that, we got along really well.

He sent me a card one time that I think summed up our relationship well. It said "Older Siblings" on the front of the card, and when you opened it up it said, "Creating trust issues since forever." I can't blame him, I tormented him growing up. I say it was all in good fun, I'm not sure he agrees.

Either way, he is one of the funniest people I've ever met and can make me laugh any time any day. My mom always says, "He's such a ham," because he is. She's right. Byron has all the academic skills that I never got. He is a CPA for an accounting firm now which amazes me. I absolutely hate math. I took statistics in high school just so I did not have to take calculus. I am terrible with numbers, and he is a CPA. I would never say we are complete opposites, but from that standpoint, we definitely are.

My grandparents, mom, dad, and Byron shaped who I am today. Each one of them played a critical role to me being able to say that I am living the happy, healthy life I always imagined. And, each of them did that in their own unique way.

I can thank my Granny and Pop-pop for teaching me unconditional love.

I can thank my Grandma Fran and Buddy for teaching me… "This too, shall pass," and the ability to know that if things are not okay yet, then, it's not the end.

I can thank my mom for always being the shoulder I needed to cry on and for having the uncanny ability to empathize with whatever crazy feeling I might have been having through this journey.

I can thank my dad for, well, for being like me... being stubborn and telling me the truth even when I didn't want to hear it. And then I'd thank him for always making me smile and laugh.

I can thank Byron for always being a steady and calming force in the family. When chaos was going on around Byron with my health, he was always there, providing support and love. I can only imagine how hard it is on the sibling of somebody living with a disability. Attention can unintentionally be diverted. Byron was strong and steady... through everything. He is our family's ray of sunshine on even the darkest of days.

Abby's Advice

While only one person is physically having the seizures, epilepsy affects families. Every person who loves the individual having the seizure is hurt when it happens. Don't be afraid to talk about it.

THREE

The Declaration

~~~~~~~~~~~~~~~~~~~~~~~~~~~~~~~~

"Our greatest glory is not in never falling but in rising every time we fall."

CONFUCIUS

Our schedule as a family was busy. We were always on the go. Every weekend, Byron and I had sports tournaments. My mom and I would go one way, and my dad and Byron would go the other. One weekend, Mother's Day weekend to be exact, after I had just turned 14, we ended up losing in our softball game on Saturday and had Sunday off.

It was rare, but we enjoyed our days off. A day off on Mother's Day meant we got to go out to an amazing brunch on Sunday morning. My absolute favorite restaurant growing up was Surf and Sirloin off of Manchester Road. I absolutely love that place! As a family, we would go there for almost every holiday, because it was Buddy's favorite place too.

I love that food, so of course, I left the restaurant feeling completely full, but happy I got to eat my all-time favorite meal – seafood pasta. There was always a buffet which my brother and boy cousins preferred, but I always chose my favorite dish off the menu every time. It was a treat!

We got home, and I was feeling exhausted. I wasn't sure why, but I was very tired.

I yelled on my way upstairs, "Mom, I'm going to lay down!"

I always took naps in my parents' king size bed. They had a huge bed and a nice big TV. Byron and I weren't allowed to have TVs in our rooms until college. Even then, they told me no. But it was college, and as soon as they left, I went out and bought my own!

Anyway, I went upstairs and started watching Lifetime, our favorite past time when we weren't running around from one activity to the other. I laid down and turned on the TV.

My mom came up and laid next to me.

"What are we going to watch?"

"Let's see what's on Lifetime."

"Great idea."

We started watching a movie, and within the first 20 minutes, I was asleep. I don't remember this well, but my mom does, so the account of this particular seizure is courtesy of my mom.

Shortly after I fell asleep, I had a seizure.

My head arched back violently, I gasped, and started violently shaking. My eyes rolled back in my head and I started foaming at the mouth... again. It had been two years since my mom saw my first seizure, so this was still very new.

She was terrified.

"ACE! ACE! HELP!!!"

"Abby, Abby!"

"Oh my god... DOYLE!" My mom was helpless... all over

again. What was happening?

"Not again! No, god, no! Not again!"

My dad rushed up the stairs and saw it for the first time with his own eyes. His precious daughter, his only daughter, was having a violent grand mal seizure.

My dad kneeled by my side. They had done research two years earlier to understand what happened and what to do during a seizure, but it was just that… two years ago. Seizure first-aid was not something they understood. My mom dialed 911.

"Please help! Please, come now. My daughter's having a seizure. Oh god, Doyle… help her."

"Ma'am… ma'am, you need to relax, is she still seizing?"

"Yes! Oh, Abby, Abby!!!"

"You need to turn her on her side if possible, so she doesn't swallow her tongue."

"Doyle, she said turn her on her side!!! Oh my god, she could swallow her tongue, ACE!"

"OUCH! Son of a bitch!" my dad yelled! He was not supposed to put anything in my mouth, but the potential for me to swallow my tongue triggered him to try and help me.

"Don't put anything in her mouth Doyle!!!" my mom snapped at him.

"Well, what should we do?!?"

"Oh, oh thank god, it's stopped… she's not shaking anymore."

"Okay ma'am… the paramedics are on their way. Now, you need to understand that she is going to be out of it for about 30 minutes to an hour. She will be in what's called the postictal phase, where she will be extremely disoriented from her seizure."

"Okay… the what phase???"

"The postictal phase."

"Okay… oh, ACE… I hear sirens, go get them."

The Chesterfield police arrived first, and shortly after the paramedics were there.

We went through the exact same exercises that we did the first go around. Do you know your name? Do you know what day it is?

My mom said that the paramedics arrived at the house after the seizure was over and told them that they could drive me to the hospital themselves and that I would be just fine.

She told me later, "Absolutely not. We were terrified and had no idea what was going on… you were going in the ambulance!"

Abby's Advice

The postictal phase is a scary phase of the seizure. If it's a tonic-clonic or grand mal seizure like I have, the convulsions have stopped and that is when the postictal phase starts. During this phase, a person is typically very disoriented. They may not be able to talk or walk. Personally, I never can. The duration of this phase varies from person to person, but usually it lasts anywhere from 30 minutes to an hour.

Shortly after I arrived (in the ambulance) to the Emergency Room, I 'came to' in a hospital bed at St. Luke's right down the street from my parent's house on Appalachian Trail. I didn't 'come to' on my second seizure like I did on my first. This piece of my journey is very blurry for me. I remember waking up briefly in the Emergency Room at St. Luke's, but I do not remember any conversations that we had or any of the tests that I had.

I was resting with IVs in a fresh hospital gown on, and suddenly… BAM! Another seizure.

My head arched back, my eyes rolled back in my head and my body was rigid. I was having seizure number two within hours of the first on Mother's Day of my freshman year of high school.

My parents pushed the button for help and started screaming "HELP!" to the nurses and doctors in the emergency room. They upped the anti-convulsant medication that was coming through my IV to help me.

I can say now the fact that I had two seizures so close together that day is probably why this particular piece of my story is so blurry.

After the second seizure that day, the ER doctors had Dr. Nicklaus, my pediatric neurologist from two years earlier, paged. They wanted him involved now. After the second seizure that day, things got serious. I was admitted for an overnight stay and would stay there until the next morning until we could figure things out.

Dr. Nicklaus showed up bright and early the next morning. My parents stayed with me at the hospital. I have no recollection of our conversation that next morning. But, my mom told me she remembers distinctly what he said.

"Abby's declared herself," Dr. Nicklaus said.

She said those words will forever be burned in her brain. He meant, on Mother's Day in 1997, I declared myself an epileptic.

"We are going to keep her here for monitoring until the end of the day, then, release her. In the meantime, I'm starting her on Trileptal, an anti-convulsant medication. She'll need doses in the morning and at night. We know Depakote did not work for her, so we will try something different this time."

He took out his prescription pad and wrote my mom the prescription right then and there and handed it to her. He shook both my mom's and my dad's hand and said I'll see you later this week.

Little did I know at that point, I was in for a lot of doctors' appointments over the next few months, and even years.

THE DIAGNOSIS

We went back to Dr. Nicklaus to get the official diagnosis later that week.

Walking back in to Dr. Nicklaus's, aka the Professor's office, was a sad day. I knew what the medicine he prescribed to me the first time did to my body, so I could only hope and pray I was not going to go down that path again. Luckily for me, we weren't going anywhere near Depakote again. This time, we would test out Trileptal.

Once again, my mom and I sat with Dr. Nicklaus, recapping what happened. Luckily, he knew most of it since he had just met us in the hospital days before.

Just as I had last time, I sat and listened to my mom explain everything.

He leaned back in his chair casually as he asked questions about my health since my very first seizure. He listened to my mom explain everything, in grave detail, that happened when I was on Depakote. He listened to her concerns about Trileptal that she was already having. It did not take long for that medication to have similar effects on me.

When I say he listened to everything this time, I mean he

listened to her talk about all of the negative effects of the medicine. We talked about how it had effected my school work, how it had effected my lifestyle and in turn, my family's lifestyle.

As he listened, I could tell he was thinking. He looked like he was thinking very hard. Finally, Dr. Nicklaus straightened up. He leaned over his big mahogany desk, put his hands together on his desk and looked at both of us.

"You have epilepsy, Abby."

Abby's Advice

How is a person diagnosed with epilepsy and what is it?

A person is typically diagnosed with epilepsy after they have had at least two seizures. In most cases, the cause is unknown, although some people develop epilepsy as a result of a brain injury or other medical condition. It's a neurological disorder that affects the nervous system, specifically the brain. According to the Epilepsy Foundation, "Seizures are caused by disturbances in the electrical activity of the brain."

"Okay," I said slowly. "So, what does that mean?"

He explained epilepsy is a seizure disorder. He explained simply that a grand mal seizure, which is what I had, happens when "the brain is trying to send too many messages at one time" to simplify things for me.

He explained that it's also referred to as a tonic-clonic seizure. A tonic-clonic or grand mal seizure has some very distinct characteristics, he nodded his head toward my mom because she had already seen those characteristics.

He explained that my muscles stiffened. He explained that the reason I don't remember any of what happens is because I am unconscious. He said your arms and legs jerk rapidly and sometimes violently. You may or may not bite your cheek and/or tongue when it happens, and you may drool or have a little foam around your mouth. The seizures typically tend to last anywhere from one to three minutes.

"Oh, jesus… it feels like way longer than that!"

I looked over at my mom with the death stare that only a teenage girl can perfect. I was thinking, seriously, mom?!?

Dr. Nicklaus, smiled, and replied, "Yes. When somebody starts having a tonic-clonic seizure, it definitely feels longer than that."

He looked back at me, "Do you have any questions about everything I've just told you?"

I had a million, but I could think of zero. I was so in shock by everything he had just told me, that I wanted to cry. Why me?

"I'd like to run a few more tests as soon as possible, the most important being a sleep deprived EEG. I'll have you stay up until midnight and wake up at 4 A.M. and start the test at 8 A.M. You will likely fall asleep during the test, so we can try to get a reading and see what is going on," Dr. Nicklaus said.

"My goal is to try to treat this with medicine, but that doesn't always work. People with epilepsy often have breakthrough seizures. We just have to play with dosage, see your limitations, see your thresholds, and go from there."

Huh? I'm thinking to myself, so I will be on anti-seizure meds, but you as my doctor are telling me that they might not work???

And what do you mean by play with dosage?

The shock never wore off long enough for me to ask any relevant questions.

I walked out of Dr. Nicklaus' office that day with three distinct thoughts...

1) I have epilepsy, what does that even mean?

2) What do I do if I have another one?

3) There is no cure for this disorder.

Two of the three were questions with no answers. And the one answer we did have was that this was not going away.

Abby's Advice

Questions for the doctor when you or a loved one are first diagnosed:

- How do you determine what dosage of medicine to give me?
- What are the treatment options before we just try medicine?
- Will I know when a seizure is coming?
- What should I do if I'm alone?
- What tests do you plan to run to help us better understand the disorder?
- How often do you want to see me?
- How often are we going to check my medication levels?
- What side effects can I expect?

ULTIMATE BETRAYAL

All of the tests Dr. Nicklaus ran came back inconclusive. We were not able to determine a root cause of the seizures. He was never able to "capture" me having a seizure during the EEG. Therefore, it was difficult to give us any information at all.

I had multiple breakthrough seizures on Trileptal (on top of feeling terrible), he quickly switched me over to Tegretol.

My quality of life was slowly dwindling. There were many times throughout my sophomore and junior year that my parents (and I) could tell this disorder was starting to affect my life beyond just the physical seizure itself.

I played softball and soccer, but soccer was my absolute favorite. It was a custom for the Varsity soccer team to have a sleepover before the season started every year. By the Spring of my sophomore year, my seizures were unpredictable. We (as a family) could not predict when or where the next one would happen.

I would do really well for four to five months, and then I'd have a really bad seizure. I would sometimes fall out of bed or bite my tongue, or worse, both. And, I would be miserable for a few days. Needless to say, our family was on edge.

My parents decided that year they did not want me to go to the annual soccer sleepover, because of the fear that I would either have a seizure at the party or be so tired from the lack of sleep that I would have one shortly thereafter. I knew I was different, but I was not okay with that. When they told me no, I could not go, I was devastated.

I remember crying alone in my room, because all the girls

would get to have so much fun without me. They would all bond without me. It was an awful feeling, to say the least. But, no matter how much of a fight I put up, my parents made their decision. I was not going.

I'll never forget waking up the Saturday morning *after* the "soccer sleepover." My family and I woke up and our house had been toilet papered. My so-called "friends," the girls who I thought understood why I couldn't go in the first place, had just TP'd our house. It was a sea of white at our house on Appalachian Trail.

I started crying. I felt betrayed by my "friends." I thought to myself, do they think I didn't come to the sleepover because I didn't want to? Why would they do this to me? That's just so mean of them. It was mean girl bullying at its finest. I was devastated and so hurt by what they did to me that night and will never forget it.

I ache for people who get bullied. Believe me, I've been there. It's a helpless and lonely feeling. To people who are victims of bullying, I promise that one day, living through that, will make you a stronger person if it hasn't already.

Abby's Advice

"True forgiveness is when you can say, 'Thank you for that experience.'" – Oprah

To the girls that TP'd me that night, thank you. I learned one thing from that night, be kind. No exceptions. One in 26 people in the United States will develop epilepsy at some point in their lifetime, I hope you will be kind to the next person that crosses your path.

ONE STEP BEHIND

Manipulating the medicine was starting to have little, if any, impact on if I'd have another seizure. I'd do fine for a period of time and then would have another seizure.

I tried to keep up with the high level sports I was playing, but it was difficult. I'm not sure if it was the medicine or the breakthrough seizures I kept having. I think it was probably a combination of both.

Up to this point, all my life, I was a soccer all-star. I was on the Missouri Olympic Development Team (ODP). I played select soccer for J.B. Marine, but by late sophomore and early junior year, I was always about one step off during the games. I played in the sweeper position, and I loved it. Playing defense was so much fun for me, but unfortunately, as the last line of defense, you cannot afford to be one step off. You have to be one step ahead… always, so the other team doesn't get a shot on goal. I always was, too… prior to this period of time.

The unmatched ball skills, speed, and coordination I always seemed to have were just "off" enough to the point where the coaches had no other option but to take me out of the starting lineup. I went from a starter to a sub within a year.

On top of being benched, my parents (and I) were worried about me doing head balls in the games. Defensive players head the ball a lot, especially when the offense has a corner kick. It's often the only way to clear the ball so the other team doesn't get a shot on goal.

Of course, my family and I did not know what was causing

my seizures, so any type of potential head injury scared us. Moral of the story, I did not need to be out on the soccer field clearing any more corner kicks. I needed to take extra special care of my head and my brain.

My dad ended up talking to the coach without my knowledge. In hindsight, it was probably a really good thing. During that time period, I only got to play in the games when the team was not concerned with the outcome. I did not understand why at the time or know that my coaches were concerned for my health too. It wasn't just my parents.

They knew my skills were better than what I was offering, but they knew something wasn't right, and so did I. Accepting the fact that being an all-star soccer player was probably not in the cards for me, I focused on other activities at school. It worked too. I fell in love with student council.

I focused on being the President of our class Senior year instead of sports. Becoming the President afforded me the opportunity to emcee our school's Homecoming pep rally and speak at our Graduation. Those two opportunities meant way more to me than any game I ever played.

Speaking at my high school graduation was definitely a high point for me. While nerves got the best of me right before I walked on stage, the speech was a success. I, for the life of me, can't remember what I said or the message that I talked about, but I do remember how I felt in that moment. I felt proud of what I had accomplished in high school and excited about my future. It was an amazing day.

Just like anybody else, high school for me had its ups and downs. Epilepsy definitely affected my social life, but I would honestly say, my experience as a whole was mostly positive. I look back on those years fondly knowing what all we went through as a family and how difficult those four years actually were.

As President, during Homecoming week, I was responsible for making sure our class float was complete and looking presentable for the day of the big game. That was always really fun for me, and I had a great group of friends supporting the effort.

Many of the friends that I made in high school, shockingly enough, are still close friends of mine today… not so much the ones who betrayed me so hurtfully the night of the sleepover, but others. I know that is probably hard for some people to believe, but it's kind of "one of those things" unique to St. Louis. Many people who grew up there, stay there. On top of that, if you leave, you usually end up going back at some point.

Personally, I do not have any intentions of doing that, because I love Houston, but I've learned over time to never say never.

Abby's Advice

"I was smart enough to go through any door that opened." - Joan Rivers

Always remember that when one door shuts, another one opens. When you have seizures, it may feel like all the doors around you are shutting. Just remind yourself, that's when another one will open. That's what happened for me. I found other passions that ultimately made me much happier.

TEARDROPS

Seizure medications are extremely sensitive. The side effects are intense on one hand, but on the other hand, if you don't take them religiously it's likely that your body will react by having a seizure. At least, that's what happens to me. Every. Single. Time.

My parents and I constantly battled throughout my sophomore and junior years of high school about me taking my medicine. For some reason, I just never saw it as important as they did. I think a lot of it had to do with the fact that I never saw myself have a seizure.

They were always the ones who had to watch me and care for me afterwards. I understand now, as an adult, how emotional watching someone you love have a seizure can be, but in high school, I had absolutely no appreciation for it.

This story is courtesy of my mom, and it is one that has stuck with me forever. She told me this story one day when she was begging me to take my medicine on time.

THUD!

"ACE!! ACE!!! It's Abby!!! Go get her!" My mom said this as she shook my dad awake.

"Oh geez! Did she just fall out of bed?! It's okay... I'll go!!" he said as he jumped out of bed.

My dad raced down the hall into my bedroom. I had just fallen out of bed and was having another grand mal seizure. My dad kneeled down next to me, picked up my rigid body and turned me on my side. He stayed with me until the seizure passed. My mom followed shortly behind him and stood in the doorway of my bedroom. She was terrified and standing there in her nightgown.

She watched with her arms crossed, hand up to her mouth, eyes wide and frightened.

After about two minutes, my body relaxed. My dad wiped the drool from my mouth and his arm, and he lifted me back up in bed. He placed my head down gently on my pillow and covered me up with my comforter. My mom walked over and they stood over me as I lay there sleeping.

They both kissed me on the forehead and headed back to bed. There was nothing more they could do for me. I needed to sleep.

At this point, my family and I had lost count of the number of seizures I had had. There were too many to count.

He grabbed my mom's hand, and they walked back to their bedroom and laid down in complete darkness.

My mom recounted this story for me later, and her words to me about the aftermath of this particular seizure are chilling.

"Abby, you don't know what it's like to watch you have a seizure. You don't understand how traumatizing it is! If you'd just take your medicine on time, this won't happen!!!

We are begging you to just take your medicine, so you don't keep having seizures!" I could tell her patience with me and the situation was wearing thin.

"I don't like my medicine! I don't like the way it makes me feel! So, I don't care!!" I screamed. My patience with the medicine and feeling "off" was wearing thin too.

"You don't care?? You don't care??? Well, I can't do this anymore, Abby! Last night, after you had your seizure, Dad and I laid down. I heard him sniffling. I could not see him, but I heard him. I reached over and felt his cheek and tears were running down his face…" her eyes welled with tears.

I felt like I had been punched in the gut.

"Dad was crying??? Because *I* had a seizure???"

"Yes, Abby. He had tears running down his cheek. Do you know how awful that is for me?"

"Why?"

"It's so hard to watch, Abby. You don't know how hard it is to see you have a seizure. Please, I'm begging you to just take your medicine, I don't know what else to do," my mom said. We sat in silence as I tried to digest the enormity of what she had just confided in me.

"Okay. I'll take it."

I could not believe it. I literally could not believe it. I had never seen my dad cry. I'm still not even sure if "tears running down your cheeks" is crying, but that was his version of it. Somehow, at that moment, it sounded worse to me than a good solid cry. And, that moment stuck with me forever.

I did not want to be the reason for my family's angst, I still don't. That's not fair to them. I started taking my medicine religiously after that day.

Unfortunately, for me and for my family, I was still having breakthrough seizures. My turning point was not as effective as we would have liked it to be. At this point, I had tried three different medications, and I was still having breakthrough seizures that were 100 percent unpredictable. We needed help.

Abby's Advice

To parents:

Talk to your teenager. Chances are, they are completely oblivious to how their disorder is affecting you. They probably don't want to hear it, but they need to. Help them understand the emotional turmoil that you go through each time you see them have a seizure. When I found out how it affected my family, I wanted to be part of the solution and not just the problem.

Fellow epileptics:

Yes, taking medicine is extremely frustrating. I get it. But, it's not worth a seizure. It took me a very long time to come to that, so my hope is that my honesty can get you there faster.

FOUR

The Next Step

*"You can't look back - you just have to put the past behind you,
and find something better in your future."*

JODI PICOULT

I did not want to have seizures anymore, and Tegretol was not working either. As a family, we were frustrated. We scheduled another follow up with Dr. Nicklaus. Before we went in, he asked that we do one more sleep deprived EEG.

I'll never forget it either. I had to stay up until midnight and wake up at 4 A.M. and go to the EEG test at 8 A.M.

Staying up until midnight was pretty easy for me. I was a night owl in high school. I preferred nights to mornings. Waking up at 4 A.M. back then was miserable. These days, 5:30 A.M. and I'm up and at 'em!

As she always was back then, my mom was right there with me. Both my dad and my mom stayed up with me until midnight. They were not as much fun as my friends were, so it was a little harder not to doze off as we watched movies, but I managed. I headed up the stairs to my bedroom and was out immediately. At

4 A.M. sharp, I felt my mom gently nudge my shoulder.

"Time to wake up!"

"No… go away," I said and rolled over to face away from her.

"You have to get up now. Come on, you only have to be up for a couple hours, and you can go right back to sleep," she said with the patience only a mom can understand. "Let's go downstairs."

I was groggy, but rolled over to the edge of the bed. I swung my legs around, and sat slumped over ready to fall back asleep at a moment's notice. My mom grabbed both of my hands, and lifted my entire body up quickly in one fast motion, so I didn't have time to change my mind. I was up. I was half asleep, but I was on my feet.

"Ready??"

"Yep, let's go. I'm up now," I said as I rolled my eyes.

The house was still pitch black. My mom was in her nightgown, and I was in my pajamas, juicy sweatpants and a faded old soccer tournament T-shirt. I remember wearing those sweatpants to bed, because I was frustrated at the situation. My dad hated those sweatpants. He didn't understand that *Juicy* was a brand, not just some word I liked on my pants. I realize now just how hard I made my parents lives back then. Every little thing to rebel, I pretty much did it.

We made the trek down the stairs and turned on all the lights to help us stay awake. There's not much going on at 4 A.M., so my mom sat in the chair directly in front of the TV in the family room and flipped it on.

I sat right across from her on the couch.

"What should we watch?" she asked me.

"I have no idea what's even on at this hour of the day," I mumbled. It would be really helpful if doctors could recommend a couple activities for patients when they ask them to get up this early.

My mom was channel surfing. There really was nothing on TV. As she surfed, I did everything I could to keep my eyes open. They felt so heavy. I felt helpless against my urge to sleep. I was back asleep before I knew it.

"Abs, Abs, wake up!"

My eyes wondered up to meet hers, "I'm so tired, though."

"I know you are, but you have to stay awake."

A couple minutes later, I dozed off again.

"Abby... stay awake!"

My head popped up! Eyes wide open. "Okay... I'm up... again."

Moments later... I was back asleep. Waking up at 4 A.M. was really, really hard for me. I am not going to lie. When you have nothing to do except sit there and watch TV that early in the morning, it's nearly impossible to stay awake.

This time, my mom just started laughing.

"Abby... you have to stay awake," she said as she was laughing at me. "Come on! You have to at least try! You are not even trying!"

I started laughing too, "I am trying! It's just so hard. This just seems so stupid!"

"I know, but let's just do it and get it over with."

From that moment on, I was awake... right up until my 8 A.M. EEG where they put me in the most comfortable leather recliner ever and asked me to fall asleep.

No problem!

Abby's Advice

"Sometimes crying or laughing are the only options left, and laughing feels better right now." –Veronica Roth

Take a shower and save watching a really good movie that you know will help you stay awake for the morning of your sleep deprived EEG. Any activity will work to be honest. Just have something to do. It could be baking a cake or arts and crafts, but do something! Waking up at 4 A.M. to turn on the TV and channel surf was a huge mistake.

FRUSTRATION BOILS OVER

We were hoping for the best, but we were slowly learning to manage our expectations. It felt like every time we thought I was getting "better," I'd have a breakthrough seizure, which I know a lot of people can relate to.

Once again, my mom and I found ourselves in Dr. Nicklaus' big office. He greeted us with a smile and a handshake as he always did. He showed us our seats, where we had been many times before and walked around to his desk and sat down across from us.

He opened up my manila folder, and this time, he looked at both my mom and me.

"I've reviewed your results from the sleep deprived EEG. Your brain activity is normal. I'm not seeing any abnormal activity that would help us. My recommendation is to keep you on Tegretol and up the dosage to test your thresholds. We know that the dosage you are currently taking is not enough, because you are still having breakthrough seizures for unknown reasons. So, I think that's the best path forward for now."

More medicine? Seriously? That's our only option? Tegretol, in my mind, was only slightly better than Depakote. I was still sleeping way more than all of my friends. One distinct memory that I have (and so does my mom) where we both kind of realized my lifestyle was different from Tegretol was when we were at a soccer tournament.

We had a really early morning game and a late afternoon game. It was decided before the games that day that we would all go to one of my teammates houses in between games to hang out. There were about five of us. The early morning game caused all of us to be tired, so we all went to take naps as soon as we got back to my teammates house. All of the girls woke up to hang out and watch a movie, but me. I could not wake up to do that. My body needed more sleep. I slept the entire day until we had to go to the next game.

That day, I remember thinking, if they all got up to hang out and watch a movie, and I could not do that, something about this isn't right.

And, here I was, being told by a doctor that I need even more medicine than I'm on right now? I'll turn into a complete zombie. There aren't enough hours in the day for me to sleep that much. I felt defeated.

My mom looked up at Dr. Nicklaus, "Are there any other medicines that you think we should try with Abby? I'm not sure she can afford to take more medicine Dr. Nicklaus. She sleeps all the time. We've noticed over the past months, she sleeps a lot more than her friends, just from the different activities they all do together and from talking to people."

"We could, but I'd recommend a higher dosage before we just move away from Tegretol."

My feelings of being mad had passed. I had moved on to a feeling of defeat.

I think it's safe to say we both walked out of the doctor's office that day with our heads down. We were told that day, for the first time, I don't know and the only recommendation that was given to us, was to take more medicine.

As we were driving home, I said to my mom, "I feel like Dr. Nicklaus didn't care today. It felt like he was just done with me, like he does not want to try to figure out why I'm having seizures… and I really don't want to take more medicine on top of that."

"I kind of felt that exact same way."

I welled up in the car with my mom as she pulled up to the bank.

"Mom, I don't want to have seizures anymore. I don't like the way I feel. I just don't want to have these anymore."

"I know, Abby. I'm sorry. I don't want you to have them either."

She leaned over to hug me, and I cried harder. "I just want to be normal again, to feel normal again."

"I know. It'll be okay. We will figure this out together."

We both realized that day that it was time to move on from Dr. Nicklaus. Epilepsy for adolescents was never his focus. His pediatric neurology practice focused on ADHD. Yes, he was considered one of the very best pediatric neurologists, and I still believe he is. I really think, and still do to this day, that he felt like he had exhausted all his options. He did not want to leave us high and dry, but at the same time, that day he kind of made it clear without saying the words, he'd done all he knew to do for me.

It was time to see somebody who dealt with children and teens with epilepsy all the time.

Abby's Advice

Because there is no cure for epilepsy, I think finding a doctor is difficult. One-third of all people with epilepsy live with uncontrollable seizures because no available treatments work for them. Those people ultimately have to trust what doctors say and what they prescribe, and no matter what, you still *could* have a seizure. It makes for a trying process.

Try to find a doctor that specializes in seizures and epilepsy. In this day and age, there are plenty of really great neurologists and epileptologists to see. I believe it will make a difference for you or your loved one in the long run if you find one you feel really understands or cares about your quality of life.

FIVE

In Pursuit of Answers

"Faith is taking the first step even when you don't see the whole staircase."

DR. MARTIN LUTHER KING JR.

It was time to see a specialist. I say we needed to see a specialist now, but at the time, I didn't know where to start. After that last visit with Dr. Nicklaus, I knew we needed to make a change, but had no idea that there were epilepsy specialists. My parents were the driving force to getting me where I needed to be.

Luckily for my family and me, St. Louis has one of the most reputable Children's hospitals in the country. They provide extraordinary care to children with disabilities and disorders of all types. The Epilepsy Center at St. Louis Children's Hospital, in partnership with the Washington University School of Medicine, has one of the largest epilepsy clinics in the world.

After extensive research and consultations with people all over the U.S., they decided that I was going to start seeing Dr. Palmer. Within the pediatric neurology community, he is one of the best. He has been recognized nationally, and it's no surprise why. Some of his research in patients with epilepsy is funded by the National Institutes of Health.

Even though I knew it was time to move on from Dr. Nicklaus, I remember looking at my dad with tears and asking him, "Why do I have to see another doctor?"

At that point, I had been doing really well. I was on what my family and I like to call "a good stretch."

He looked at me and stated, "Because he's the best, Abby. *That* is who we are going to see."

I was not about to continue asking him why. He made that statement in a very matter of fact tone, and what I had to say about it was not going change the fact that I was headed downtown to St. Louis Children's Hospital.

THE EPILEPSY CENTER AT CHILDREN'S

The first time I walked in to the waiting room at Epilepsy Center at Children's, I had all kinds of emotions.

I was impressed. It was huge compared to the waiting room at Dr. Nicklaus' office. It was also very friendly and inviting. There were toys everywhere. As a high schooler, I was not interested in those, but I could see where that type of environment would be nice for a kid. Kids were playing with blocks, reading books, and wondering around the waiting room to different toy stations.

I was scared. There were kids in the same waiting room as me that looked and were significantly more disabled than I was. I knew epilepsy was considered a disability, but many of the kids were wearing helmets and some were wheelchair bound. It was eye opening.

I started to feel annoyed, why did I need a specialist? My dad's answer of "he is the best" was a distant memory once I stepped foot in that room. That day, I was not grasping the seriousness of the situation. Each and every person with epilepsy is only one serious seizure away from being wheelchair bound.

I was frustrated. Missing school and taking a full day off to go to a doctor seemed excessive. Why were my parents dead set on me seeing this doctor?

Most of the feelings I had that day were negative. All those feelings combined came out in one single form… anger. I was angry that I had this damn epilepsy and I was angry I needed to be there in the first place.

I wish I could have controlled my anger a little that day. Now I look back and can't believe how many people were in that same waiting room as me waiting to be treated for the same disorder. I finally found the other people I was looking for. I was constantly wondering where all the "other" people with epilepsy were. I would think to myself, how is it that one in 26 people have epilepsy? That has to be a lie. I don't know anybody!

As I sat there and pondered that fact and why I still had not actually *met* anybody else with seizures, the nurse came and called my name. My mom and I walked back while the nurse held the door open. She took my height and weight right there in the hallway on our way back to the patient room. The room was small with an exam table on the right with two chairs directly across from it. I hopped on the exam table and my mom took a seat in one of the chairs across from me.

The nurse quickly took my vitals, said everything looked good.

"The doctor will be in shortly," she said as she left the room.

I looked at my mom and gave her a half smile.

"How are you feeling?" my mom asked.

"Fine, I guess."

"When he comes in, do you want to talk?"

"I guess."

"I think you should. It would be good for him to hear from you."

I shrugged my shoulders and didn't respond. I just stared at the white walls. It was a much friendlier room than the rooms I've been in since then as an adult, but it was still very white.

After the nurse took my vitals, I became overwhelmed with so many emotions that I did not really know how to respond to my mom asking me questions. In that moment, for whatever reason, I shut down. All the emotions I was having left me speechless. The high and low emotions overpowered me. I was already a teenage girl, and then to add this to the mix, it left me feeling beat down in that moment.

When I was at Dr. Nicklaus' office, all I wanted was for him to ask me about how I felt and ask me the questions. I was having flashbacks of how frustrated I felt when he would look at my mom and ask her everything the whole time we met.

Now, I was about to have the opportunity to answer and talk and provide feedback, and all I could say when my mom asked me if I wanted to talk was, "I guess" in a nonchalant, irritated manner.

She knew how frustrated I was that doctors were asking her about my disease. And, yet, there we were, sitting there about to talk to one of the most well-respected epilepsy doctors in the entire country, probably the world, and I was pissed off about being in that white room and in turn, fell silent.

We both looked at the door as soon as we heard the three light knocks at the door. In walked Dr. Palmer. My first impression was that he looked young and also that he looked smart.

He looked at me first and introduced himself.

"Abigail, I'm Dr. Palmer… Nice to meet you."

What a nice change of pace is what I was thinking! I mustered, "Hi."

We shook hands.

Instantly, I felt a little more comfortable. "Please call me Abby."

Now, I look back and wonder why I was not more excited to meet such an amazing doctor who is so well regarded in the epilepsy community. I can sum it up in a couple words, naivety, immaturity, and inexperience.

Then, he introduced himself to my mom. He sat on his stool near the desk at the back of the room and rolled over closer to us to start our conversation. He already had my files from Dr. Nicklaus' office, so he knew why we were there.

He had his manila folder with all of my information in it, opened it to the first page and started talking.

"So, you have epilepsy… can you tell me a little bit about what you've experienced so far?" He was looking at me when he asked the question. But, rather than seize that opportunity and take advantage of everything that I wanted to say, I looked at my mom with the… hello, this-is-your-turn-to-answer face.

She looked at me with big eyes, as in, are you seriously not going to respond?

It was true… I wanted her to re-hash everything.

He was turned toward me when he asked the first question, but quickly swiveled to give my mom and her explanation his full attention.

She detailed my first seizure. She detailed my second and third seizures. She detailed our appointments with Dr. Nicklaus. She detailed every medication I had taken to that point, the name, the dosage, what time I took it.

I know every person with seizures is different, but I have always taken a small dose in the morning to get me through the day, and a heftier dose at night… no matter what drug… because I'm prone to seizures while I am sleeping.

My mom explained to Dr. Palmer, at that point we had tried Depakote, Trileptal, and Tegretol. All three of these medications put me into a zombie-like state. It took us, as a family, a good two and a half years to try all those different medications and to find Dr. Palmer. By the time we were sitting there in his office that day, I felt like I had lost a good chunk of my high school years to sleep.

My mom talked about how I was having a hard time getting out of bed. She described how I could not concentrate at school. She spelled out for him in grave detail that she thought I was feeling sad and hopeless.

Seizure medications are mood and lifestyle altering drugs. Just like I cringe when I hear that people are still taking Depakote, I cringe at the fact that the medicines that turned me into a different person are still being used to treat seizures today and its nearly 20 years later. I know that is not the best this country, with the amazing doctors and the amazing technology we have at our fingertips, can do.

Dr. Palmer swiveled his chair to look at me now.

"Are those things true? Tell me about that."

It was time for me to open up.

"I feel tired all the time. I think I look sad and hopeless, because I'm so tired and drowsy. I don't think I'm sad, but I know I'm tired. I could sleep on this table if you gave me a pillow."

"Okay. Okay. I understand."

Dr. Palmer was very patient and friendly. He looked down and looked to me like he was thinking very hard about what steps to take next.

He looked up, looked at my mom, and then looked at me.

"I have a few recommendations."

Dr. Palmer explained that the medicines I was taking were not medicines that doctors in the epilepsy community would consider the latest and greatest drugs. New anti-convulsant drugs were introduced to the market that he would like me to try. We could start my weening me off of Tegretol, all while I would start taking Keppra.

After briefly discussing the medicines and how we would be changing it up, which gave me great relief, he asked us a question that I will never forget.

This question has been one that I've thought about over and over because it literally changed my life.

"How do you feel about us doing a video EEG?"

I looked at my mom, she looked back at me, and we looked together at him.

"What is that?" we asked in perfect sync.

I cannot remember in detail how he explained it, but I'm going to take the opportunity to explain it how I prefer.

In summary, you are put in a room, hooked up to a computer

with a bunch of electrodes all over your head for multiple days and videotaped 24 hours a day. The purpose of the test is to make sure you have a seizure so that the doctors can document everything.

Dr. Palmer would use all the data captured on the computer and all the footage captured on video camera to help us determine the cause of my seizures.

This would, in turn, help us figure out how to best treat them. He explained that it was a possibility if we could locate and pinpoint the exact spot in my brain that the seizures were originating from, we might be able to remove that piece, and get rid of the seizures altogether.

After Dr. Palmer detailed this procedure, my heart stopped. I looked at him.

"How in the world… no wait, why in the world would you want me to purposely have seizures?"

I was so mad. No, I was furious. This doctor was suggesting that I have seizure after seizure so he could gather data?!?

I'll be 100 percent honest. I did not see this as a solution to a problem. I did not see this as something to give my family hope. I did not see this as a way for us to get rid of my seizures.
I had one feeling, and one feeling only… I was Dr. Palmer's lab rat.

My case was complicated at that point. No doctors could figure out why I was having seizures, so he was going to save the day.

It was obvious, he and I were not going to see eye to eye on this one.

FAMILY "DISCUSSIONS"

I didn't make eye contact with my mom or Dr. Palmer for the rest of the doctor's visit. I was laser focused on the fact that a doctor wanted to induce seizures. The thought of this made me physically ill.

"We need to talk about this, Abby."

"Talk about what?" I was looking out the window of my mom's car on the way home from Children's and had no intentions of making eye contact with my mom knowing that she was even considering me doing this.

"The video EEG that Dr. Palmer just told us about."

"Video EEG, huh... so that's what he is calling this," I replied.

"This test could give us a lot of information that we do not have right now."

"Please don't talk to me."

As a teenager it is really hard to describe your feelings. I think it's difficult to talk about how you are feeling to your parents, and it's even more difficult to talk about your feelings to a doctor that you hardly know.

I wish that day that I would have been able to tell my mom so many things. First off, this proposition scared me. So many bad things can happen when you have a seizure. Second, was there nothing else we could try before we made that leap?

It literally felt like we went from zero to 100 in less than 60 seconds.

We got home that night and were sitting together in the family room. I was sitting on the couch with my mom and my dad was across the room in his chair.

"So tell me about your visit today," my dad said.

"Abby? Can you tell Dad about our visit?"

"Sure. It's simple. Dr. Palmer wants to turn me in to his own personal lab rat. He wants to induce seizures by taking me off my medicine and keeping me up all hours of the night..."

My mom stopped me. "Okay, let's talk this through. None of the tests we have done to date have been able to tell us anything about what causes your seizures. We still do not know why you are having seizures or what part of your brain they are originating from.

Dr. Palmer is offering to help us get those answers. The video EEG is a way for us to learn so much more about your seizures. We could treat them and possibly get rid of them completely if we could answer those questions."

I looked up at my dad for protection.

"So, tell me about this test."

My mom stepped in, and I just rolled my eyes.

"Abby would be admitted to the hospital for approximately a week. She would have an EEG, just like the ones we have already had, but it would be continuous until she had seizures. We would see the brainwaves normally and also when she is having a seizure. The electrodes would pick up that brain activity. Dr. Palmer also videotapes her in the bed having the seizure. Her movements and sounds can help him determine what region of her brain the seizures are originating from."

"What's his ultimate goal?"

"He believes that Abby has the potential to be a great candidate for brain surgery. If he can pinpoint where her seizures are originating, which he believes he might be able to using this test, then she is a surgery candidate."

I watched my mom explaining all the information we heard that day. I watched my dad processing all the information we heard that day. I was listening to all the information we heard that day… again. This time, I was actually hearing the details of how this would work and the possibilities of a seizure free future.

I jumped in. "So he really believes that brain surgery would just get rid of my seizures?"

Now that I settled down, the possibility sort of excited me.

"Yes." My mom answered with a smile.

"Well, it sounds like something that we need to move forward with to me," my dad replied.

My excitement was short-lived. The possibility of living seizure-free was no longer exciting considering what I had to go through to get there.

"I do not want to do all those tests."

Looking back, I wish I could have articulated better what I was thinking. But, at the time, it just turned in to a fight.

I'll never forget the words that ended that argument and told me all I needed to know. It was the same answer he had when we first talked about going to see Dr. Palmer in the first place.

"He's the best, Abby. He's one of the top neurologists in the country, not just St. Louis, the United States," my dad said as he got up from his chair and walked out of the room.

Tears welled up in my eyes, and I ran up the stairs to my room.

My mom followed me.

That night, whether she understood how I was feeling or

not, she listened. She didn't judge me for being upset and mad about having to do a video EEG.

She sat with me, hugged me, and let me cry it out. My mom stayed with me, she was compassionate and understanding.

Having a seizure is emotional, and at this moment in time, knowing seizures were in my near future, I cried. I cried hard. Luckily for me, my mom was there.

Abby's Advice

Write down what you are feeling and why in situations like these. This will help you formulate questions and articulate your concerns. It's okay to tell your loved ones and your doctor how you are feeling. I was never able to articulate why I felt so mad. So, keep a notebook and write it down. It will help you sort through those emotions.

WHAT IF?

We were back in the waiting room at Children's before I knew it for our pre-test to "the test."

This appointment with Dr. Palmer was to go over all the information again, get us details about the hospital stay, and answer any last minute questions we might have.

It seemed like every person in that office knew why we were there and was excited for us that day. When we walked in the receptionist greeted us in a friendlier manner.

The nurses were always nice, but this time, she looked right at me and said, "Are you excited?"

I looked at her like she was crazy. Then, I turned around and looked at my mom with a face that screamed, is this lady insane?!? This group of people obviously had seen some success with this type of testing. Having this test in their eyes was one step closer to eliminating seizures altogether.

I compare it now to a doctor doing a strep test and determining you need amoxicillin. One test, you know what medicine will cure your sore throat, and you are healed! While not the same, the concept is still relevant.

The nurses and doctors would do the Video EEG and pinpoint the origin in my brain causing the seizure. I'd have brain surgery and my seizures would be gone!

I am not going to lie, their excitement and confidence was infectious. Maybe this was going to work.

We took my height, weight, and blood pressure and walked into the exam room. My demeanor slowly started to change with the energy and confidence that Dr. Palmer and his team had. I can remember sitting in the patient room thinking to myself, what if?!

What if I did not have to take eight pills a day for the rest of my life?

What if I had the same amount of energy all of my friends have?

What if I did not have to worry about having a seizure at my next sleepover?

What if my parents never had to watch another seizure in their lives?

What if…

It was a tipping point. While up to that point, all this test had done was piss me off, I decided in that moment to change my attitude and hope that this was the answer to our prayers. No more seizures.

Dr. Palmer walked in to the patient room and greeted us. For the first time, I smiled a genuine smile at him.

He greeted us with a handshake and we all took a seat.

"I'm really glad you have decided to do Video EEG testing," he said as he looked back and forth between my mom and me.

"We are too," she replied.

I was getting excited, but I wasn't at the happy-I'm-going-through-with-this point yet.

"So, let me give you a little information about what exactly you will be doing during this week long testing.

I'm assuming a week, because it usually takes about that long for somebody to have a seizure after we have had them stop taking their medicine."

My mom and I looked at each other and we both chuckled out loud.

I actually love looking back at that moment now.

Dr. Palmer said, "What's wrong?"

I chuckled again while she explained that there was no way it was going to take a week for me to have a seizure. I could not go 12 to 24 hours without my medicine, much less a week. I thought apparently his other patients don't have as bad of epilepsy as I do.

I know that is wrong now. Epilepsy is bad no matter what. It just so happens every person's body reacts to medicine differently. My medicine is out of my system within 24 hours.

"We also want you to be sleep deprived when you come in," he stated.

We really got a kick out of that! Off medicine and sleep

deprived, there's no better formula for a seizure! It's a bad joke, but it made us laugh and eased the mood.

Dr. Palmer got us back on track and said that he understood, but it is typical that people need a week of the testing and to be sleep deprived before they can gather data.

He looked at me and said, "Abby, you've had an EEG right? So you understand what that piece is about?"

He was right. I had had an EEG with Dr. Nicklaus. The test I had with Dr. Nicklaus was easier and only a couple hours. It tracked and recorded the electrical activity in my brain while I was napping. Of course, that was the test that we learned everything looked completely normal and told us nothing.

Either way, I knew what to expect in terms of the gel-like adhesive on my scalp, the technician putting electrodes on my scalp, the test producing brain waves... yes, I got it.

"Yep," I said matter-of-factly.

"We will be adding the video component to that test. You will be in a private hospital room across the street, and there will be a camera in the corner of the room. You will have the standard electrodes on your scalp and this video on you 24 hours a day while we collect data. The information that will be most beneficial to us is the information we gather while you are having a seizure.

"There is nothing abnormal about your current EEG results, so we need to capture that disruption and the electrical activity in your brain during a seizure to understand what is going on.

"If we can do that, it will help us determine if you are a good candidate for brain surgery."

I was nervous, but said, "Okay."

I should have been prepared with questions, but I think that

I was so overwhelmed that no questions came to mind.

Mom to the rescue… "Well, I have some questions about this Dr. Palmer."

"Yes, please… shoot."

"You mentioned briefly you want Abby to be sleep deprived, and we have done that before, but what exactly are your requirements to make sure she comes in sleep deprived?" My mom was prying to see if we had to wake up at 4 A.M. again, I could tell. Neither one of us wanted to do that again!

He explained that he would like us to stay up until midnight the night before we check in to the center and wake up at six A.M. on the day we check in. Total, I would have only six hours of sleep going in to the testing. For us, that was a relief!

I looked at my mom wide-eyed, because I could not believe it! She looked at me, and said, "Don't worry, I'll be up with you," and she winked at me.

She refocused on Dr. Palmer, "When should she stop taking her medicine?"

"We do not want her to have a seizure prior to getting hooked up to the EEG and on video, so plan to take your medicine the night before, but not the morning of the test."

My mom was writing notes as he talked. It looked like she was writing down every word he said. I cannot believe back then how much I just winged it. I'm horrified now if I'm not 100 percent completely prepared for meetings at work. I guess I learned that from my mom, but that skill did not appear until adulthood.

"Will the electrodes remain attached to Abby the entire time?"

Dr. Palmer explained that I would be "wired" with EEG

electrodes during the entire stay. He explained that it's easier to wear pajamas that button or zipper down the front, and that my hair could not be washed until the electrodes were removed.

"Gross," I blurted out. "Really? I can't wash my hair at all?"

"Not during this test. I'm sorry."

"That's okay, Abs… we will figure it out."

"Any additional questions, Mrs. Gustus?"

"I think for now, I understand what we need to do, and we are ready."

"Please call me with any questions," he said to my mom.

He turned to me, "I look forward to seeing you next week, Abby."

"Oh… you will be there?"

"I'll be visiting you during your stay, yes."

"See ya then!"

He looked at my mom, "The nurse will be in shortly to get you all the details for next week."

Abby's Advice

Additional questions for the Doctor prior to your Video EEG:

- What if I don't have seizures when I'm in the hospital?
- Are there other tests that I will have while I'm there?
- How is this information different from the sleep deprived EEG?
- What is your ultimate goal for me?
- What is the timeframe for when we will see the results?
- What will happen if a seizure lasts longer than normal?
- What do I need to bring with me?
- Can I have visitors?

PREPARATIONS

"Hi Abby, how are you today?" the nurse said as she walked in and sat down next to us.

"I'm good, how are you?" I replied.

"Hi, Mrs. Gustus, I'm doing well, thanks for asking," she replied. "I want to walk you through what to expect next week if that's okay with you."

"Yep… that sounds good."

"So, first off, you've done EEGs in the past. You understand the gist of what we are going to be doing, correct?"

"I mean I think so, I'll have that gooey stuff in my hair with the electrodes attached to them. They'll monitor my brainwaves.

Dr. Palmer did just tell us that the electrodes will be on the whole time and I can't wash my hair the whole week. That's kind of gross."

"Yes, that is part of it. You will have a little box where all of the electrodes will go, you can carry that around the room, mainly to the bathroom if you need to use the bathroom, but that will be as far as you can go for the week. We recommend bringing lots of movies and books to read.

I hear you have most of your seizures at night, correct?"

"Yeah… I only have them when I'm sleeping."

"Yes. So you will want to have stuff to do while you are awake during your stay. Bring comfortable pajamas that you can change daily, that always helps.

Okay, so, back to the test… there will be a video camera mounted up in the corner of the room next to the TV. That will record all of your movements during a seizure. That information will help Dr. Palmer a lot."

"How long do you think I'll have to do this?"

"Well, we can never pre-determine when somebody will have a seizure, so it could be just a few days if you have seizures right away or it could be up to a week or week and a half while we wait for the best data," the nurse replied as she looked at me and then back to my mom.

"What's going to be done to make sure Abby is safe when she has the seizures?" my mom asked. Good question, I thought to myself. How are they going to keep me safe?

"Good question!" The nurse thought so too.

"This is a very controlled environment. Abby will be in a hospital bed with padded arm rails to keep her from hurting herself. We ask, Mrs. Gustus, that either you or your husband be with Abby at all times.

"If she starts to have a seizure, there is a button on the side of her bed that you can push and nurses will respond to help you. That button also automatically marks the EEG, so we can go back and look at the results.

It's important for me to let you know, there is safety equipment readily available in case the seizure is longer than normal."

"Okay… okay…" my mom said as she nodded her head.

I started feeling a little anxiety. This was getting real. I was going to be put into a hospital room for one purpose only… to have seizures.

"So, Dr. Palmer mentioned we should stop her medicine the night before?"

"I've spoken to Dr. Palmer, and we understand Abby is

very sensitive to her medication. Typically, we ask people not to take medicine for 24 hours. In Abby's case, like Dr. Palmer said, we are going to only ask that you not take your medicine the morning that you come in. We don't want you to have any seizures outside the controlled environment."

I thought to myself phew. I wanted to have as few seizures as possible, and the most important thing to me sounded like we needed to make sure it was on tape.

"Any final questions?"

I looked at my mom, she looked at me.

"I think I'm ready. I feel like I understand what to expect for the most part."

"You do?" My mom questioned.

"I think so… why, are you not?"

"No, I think we are ready too. Thank you so much for your time and for helping us understand the process better. We really appreciate it."

"Not a problem, feel free to call me if you think of any additional questions between now and next week! Good luck, Abby."

The next time we would walk in that hospital, I'd be off my medicine and getting hooked up for my video EEG.

I will be sharing strategies for managing and maintaining a healthy lifestyle on my blog at www.SeizeTheDayAbby.com so be sure to check my website often for updates.

SIX

Knowledge is Power

"Knowledge is power. Information is liberating.
Education is the premise of progress, in every society, in every family."

KOFI ANNAN

Luckily (or unluckily depending on how you look at the situation) for me, taking me off my medicine usually automatically causes a seizure. Dr. Palmer had us do the sleep deprivation thing, but didn't make us wake up at 4 A.M. on top of staying up late. Just being sufficiently tired was enough. He was cool about that. I'm not sure he totally believed us, and would've liked me to do the entire sleep deprived four hours of sleep, but he conceded and chose to believe us.

On the drive down to Children's the day of my hospital stay, I felt fine. I actually don't remember feeling nervous or anxious. At that point, I accepted the fact that this was something I had to do.

The doctors and nurses at the hospital recommend that you set up visits throughout your stay. I already knew my friends were coming to visit, my aunt and uncle and cousins were coming to visit, Byron would be around when he wasn't at school, and either my mom or my dad had to be with me the whole time. Knowing I was never going to be alone eased my mind.

We got to the hospital and checked in right away. The nurse on duty showed my mom and me to our room. It was a corner room that seemed very spacious to me. It was all pastel colors, light green complimented with a light peach color on the walls. Across the room under the window was a couch. That was where one of my parents would sleep for the next few days to a week.

The nurse showed us around the room.

"Here is your bathroom, it's got a shower for your guests, but you really won't be able to use it, as you know Abby."

"Yeah… I know."

Over on the side of the bed near the couch was a chair. On the chair rested a button.

"Here is the button that we want you to hit, Mrs. Gustus, when Abby has a seizure or if you think she's having an aura. We want you to hit that. It will mark the EEG system and ping a nurse to come in immediately."

She took a deep breath and looked at my mom and me. Our eyes were wide. This was our new home for the next week.

"It'll be okay. We are going to take very good care of you. Do you have pajamas that button up or a zip up that you can change in to?"

"Yes."

"Go ahead and change and get comfortable. I'm going to let the EEG technician know you are here and ready to go."

My nerves were kicking in. I was getting scared, and she sensed it.

"Relax… everything will be okay. I'll be right back."

I looked at my mom holding back tears.

"It's okay… here come on, you want your new pajamas?"

It was the one thing that kept me excited about my hospital stay. I had super cute new pajamas. Anytime my mom and I feel anxious, that's our solution. Go shopping and make sure you look good. Even if the situation sucks, at least you look good. Sometimes it gets expensive, but it's always worth it. It, still to this day, helps my mood.

I changed in to my new pajamas, they were cute and definitely put a smile on my face.

I hopped up onto the bed, and my mom put her overnight bag over in the corner and sat on the couch. Before we could say a word, in walked the technician.

"Hi, Abby!"

She was very nice and cheery.

I will say St. Louis Children's Hospital has done a fantastic job of creating a positive environment. The hospital is inviting, and the people are very nice.

"So, you've had EEGs before, right?"

"A few… yeah."

"Okay, so can I have you sit in the chair right over here while I put the electrodes on your head?"

"Sure."

She put the electrodes on carefully one by one, cold goo and all. With each electrode my clean hair got nastier.

"Ugh… I hate having this stuff in my hair," I said as I looked at my mom.

"I can tell by your face that you don't like it," my mom said as she laughed.

She finished getting me all hooked up and handed me a box with every electrode connected to it.

"This is what you will take with you if you have to get up and use the restroom, brush your teeth, or whatever. You can walk around the room with this, but that's about as far as you will get. You can see here where it's connected," she pointed to the monitoring system that was connected to the wall, "this is all the slack that you have. To get good readings, we need to make sure that your electrodes stay in place, so try to stay in bed as much as possible. I hope you brought movies!"

"Oh yeah… I brought a bunch of movies."

"Great! Well, you will see me again… I have to come in and out to make adjustments, especially after you have a seizure. The electrodes will get moved around after those, so I just come in and re-attach or adjust any that may have moved."

"Okay… sounds good… thank you," I said as she exited the room waving good bye.

I looked over at my mom, "So, what do we do now?"

She laughed, "I guess we wait."

"I guess we wait…"

CAPTURED

When you have epilepsy and know that you will probably have a seizure if you fall asleep, it's really, *really* hard to go to sleep. Having a seizure isn't natural. Nobody wants to have one. So, it was very unnatural for me to try to sleep that night knowing that could happen. I fought sleep for as long as possible with a couple movies, but it was helpless. I was tired.

I drifted off to sleep in my hospital bed that first night with my mom right next to me on the couch around midnight.

Within hours, BOOM! I had a seizure.

My mom hit the magic button and stood up next to my bed.

My body was stiff as a board and my limbs were jerking forcefully.

Instantly, a nurse was on the other side of my bed, and my mom and the nurse turned me on my side. They helped me through the seizure as best they could.

It wasn't a long one, so no additional help was needed.

My body relaxed and so did my mom and the nurse there helping her.

"Looks like we got our first seizure on camera for Dr. Palmer," the nurse said looking at my mom. "This information will be really helpful."

My mom looked at her, "I hope so."

Obviously, my body was exhausted. I think getting the first one out of the way helped everybody relax.

I woke up the next morning in a fog. I am usually always in a pretty big fog the night after a seizure. I'm out of the postictal phase by then but still lethargic and in a haze. I can typically sleep after a grand mal seizure for a day or two before I'm finally feeling normal again. So the next morning, I was barely functioning, but I do remember distinctly my first visit from Dr. Palmer.

"Knock, knock," Dr. Palmer said as he peaked his head around the corner.

I woke up, and my mom got up to shake his hand.

"Hi, Dr. Palmer," I said and smiled at him. My mouth was sore and swollen on the inside from biting my cheek and tongue during my seizure.

"Well, so it looks like you had your first seizure last night… you both said that would happen, that's pretty amazing that it happened so fast."

"We told you!" I said with a small laugh.

"Yes… yes, you did," he smiled.

"So, I'm pretty sure we captured really good data last night, but I need to review it in more detail today. I'd also like to see a couple more while you are here if possible. So, I'm going to ask that you stay if that is okay with you."

My mom looked over at me… did I want to stay and have more seizures? Nope! Was I going to because that's what my parents wanted me to do? At that point, yes.

"Great… that will only help us, and it will give us much more conclusive data if we see a few more seizures."

I was too tired from my seizure the night before to fight anything. Internally, I was frustrated at the idea of having more seizures, but I knew that's what I was there for. I was there to try and figure this out and see if I was a candidate for brain surgery. Brain surgery to cure me of this horrible disorder was the goal and the ultimate prize from all this trauma.

I watched movies and slept most of the day. I'd get up occasionally to go to the bathroom… my box with the electrodes connected to them in hand, and cord dragging behind me. It felt pathetic, but it was just part of the process that I gave in to and accepted.

My dad relieved my mom that afternoon so she could go home and rest. It's hard enough to sleep on a couch in a hospital bed, much less, when it's dependent on you that you watch for the seizure.   There's no doubt in my mind, my mom didn't sleep well when she had to just sit there and wait for a seizure.

So, my dad showed up, which was a nice change of pace. He came in that afternoon, and I was too tired to care what was on TV anymore, so I handed him the remote and let him watch whatever he wanted. I was asleep really early.

Sure enough, half way through the night on night two… another seizure.

My head turned back, my eyes rolled back in my head, I gasped and was having another full blown seizure.

My dad hit the button and the nurse was in the room with him instantly.

I had my seizure and slowly again, without any help from the nurse, my body relaxed and I drifted back to sleep. It was my second seizure within 24 hours. My body was spent.

My mom showed up early the next morning. I woke up for a brief moment when she was there. Shortly after my mom arrived, a nice (and funny) nurse came in to check all my vitals.

"Somebody hit that button last night a couple times… and hard," she said as she looked at my dad and winked. "We got the message!"

"Hell yeah, I hit that button!" my dad said.

It was hilarious… I can only imagine how many times he hit that button that you are only supposed to hit once. We all started laughing. It was one of the happy moments of my hospital stay. I'll always remember that nurse giving my dad a hard time. I just thought that was great, and it totally made my day.

Shortly after that, the EEG technician came in and adjusted my electrodes. They had moved during the seizure slightly so she fixed them. My hair was beginning to look absolutely disgusting, but there was nothing I could do about it, so I just accepted it. Plus, I was too exhausted to care.

On day two, flowers started to arrive from friends and family, so that felt really great. I had never gotten flowers before (outside of flowers for high school dances), so that was exciting. Each time I got one, my mom got up and put them on the window sill above her couch and read me the card. Day two was also the day my friends were stopping by, so that made me feel excited.

My boyfriend at the time and my friend, Laura Korbecki, who I would later end up rooming with in New York City, came to visit me. I don't remember the actual visit. I do remember them walking into the room. I remember them seeing me all wired up and the shocked and surprised looks on their faces.

They obviously had never seen somebody hooked up to an EEG before so that was a first for them. It helped a lot to have people come visit during the day. I was exhausted, but it broke it up enough so that I wasn't painfully bored.

The stay became a huge blur after the second seizure. I know I had a couple more, but I cannot recall exact timing.

I do remember Dr. Palmer coming in to talk to us about the results and what his findings were. He happened to show up at the perfect time when both of my parents were with me in the room.

My mom woke me up, so I could listen to Dr. Palmer, too.

"So, I'd like to walk through what I've learned so far from Abby's stay," he said as he started to explain the results.

Dr. Palmer backed up and explained everything. He explained that I was here in the first place because I had already "failed" five medications. That meant that even with the prescribed medicines, I was still having tonic-clonic seizures. Depakote, Trileptal, Tegretol, Keppra, and Lamictal had all failed. Dr. Palmer put me on Keppra the very first time I saw him. He added Lamictal after my first seizure on Keppra, because we felt I had hit my Keppra threshold. I was very close to that drowsy state again. It was a good combination, but I was still having breakthrough seizures. He detailed all of that to get us to where we were today.

"So, what have we learned from your stay with us here?"

He sat next to the computer and pulled up my EEG results. He showed my family and me what my brainwaves look like normally, and then he showed us what my brain waves looked like when I had a seizure. The screen went from soft green spikes and waves to a sea of green. It was amazing to look at. It was the first time I'd ever seen any data like this.

He then pulled up the video, but I said I didn't want to see it. I am so mad at myself for not watching the video of me having a seizure, but at the time, it was just too hard. I wish now, for my own knowledge, I knew what it looked like. But, in the video portion of it, Dr. Palmer learned that my head arcs back sharply to the right. That showed him that the origin point of my seizures was somewhere on the right side of my brain between my occipital and parietal lobes.

The end goal of all of this testing was to be able to pinpoint the point of origin and surgically remove that piece of my brain. But, that day Dr. Palmer explained that he could not totally define the area.

Then, Dr. Palmer dropped a bomb, "I still have to present all of our findings to the St. Louis Children's Hospital Board to get approval, but there is a chance you are a candidate for brain surgery. From the testing and with this information, there is a really big risk," he took a deep breath. "There is a 50 percent chance Abby could lose her eyesight," he said as he looked to my parents.

We all sat there in disbelief… did he just say what we think he said?

I'm not sure any of us heard much more than that, so I'm really glad he walked us through most everything else first.

I don't even remember Dr. Palmer leaving after that. Everything went blank for me that day after he said I'm a candidate for brain surgery. The surgery probably meant that my seizures would be gone forever, but with that came a 50 percent chance of going blind, which would also mean forever.

That was a lot to think about for both me and my parents.

LIFE GOES ON

I think back to these times, and it's hard to believe that life actually has to go on while all of this is happening. It was senior year of high school, and I was going away to college in the Fall. It is funny to think back on it now, because it seems like that is all we did, but it's not. We were planning for my future at the same time we were talking about having brain surgery.

I visited only two schools junior year. I was offered soccer scholarships to two smaller schools, but I never saw myself at a small university or playing a college sport for that matter. I had bigger plans… I always saw myself at a state university with tons of people!

In the Spring of my Junior year of high school, my mom forced me to go with her to visit Purdue. I expressed an interest in following in her footsteps career-wise, and Purdue had the number three program in the country for Speech Pathology. She made me visit.

I honestly have no idea why I did not want to go, but for some reason, I just didn't. It's funny to me now that I had such a strong opposition to it then. Turns out, our visit was scheduled on the most beautiful day ever. The sun was shining, and there was not a cloud in the sky. It was 75 degrees with a light breeze... just perfect!

It must have been one of the very first nice days of Spring, because college kids were outside everywhere. The campus was alive! Students were smiling. They were playing Frisbee in the Mall, and running through the fountains on campus! As we were touring, I started to feel like this might be a place I could see myself.

I was not 100 percent sure at that point, but it was definitely a possibility. After the formal campus tour and talking to students and faculty, my mom asked me to humor her and drive around.

"Just humor me, let's drive around... I'll take you by the Chi O house," she said.

I rolled my eyes and said okay.

We pulled up to Chi Omega, and she explained to me that was her sorority. She pointed out her room. Of course, at that point, I had no reference points, no real understanding of Chi Omega and so I was only about half interested. Part of me still really wanted to stay close to all of my high school friends and go to Mizzou.

It was a quick drive by, so totally painless. Afterwards, I felt happy that I had the opportunity to see where she lived when she was in college.

"Let's drive around a little, so you can get a feel for the

campus, too."

Greek life at Purdue is huge. At that point in my life, I was sure of one thing, I definitely wanted to join a sorority. I had no idea which one, but that was something that was important to me.

We pulled out onto one of the main roads close to campus. Many of the sorority and fraternity houses at Purdue are really close to campus, so it was easy to see them all.

The moment I knew I had to go to Purdue was when we drove by one fraternity house, Fiji. Tons of people were outside hanging out. Their music was blaring, and they had a water slide set up. All of the college students were playing slip 'n slide in the front yard!

This was the school for me!

I never once played slip 'n slide in college, but just the fact that I could have if I ever wanted to was enough for me to know that was going to be a really fun school. And, was. It. Ever!

I visited only two schools and applied to only two schools. There was only one, though, that had slip 'n slide. That was where I was headed.

Purdue University was a magical place for me. All of my memories there are fond. I went there not knowing a soul and left with friends for life. My sorority experience was absolutely amazing. I love those girls, and they love me. We studied, partied, then studied and partied some more. I became independent and learned a lot about myself. I'm so thankful, too, that I went out of state and out of my comfort zone.

Abby's Advice

"You have brains in your head. You have feet in your shoes. You can steer yourself any direction you choose. You're on your own. And you know what you know. And YOU are the one who'll decide where to go..." – Dr. Seuss, Oh, the Places You'll Go!

Visit many different schools. You will feel something inside your gut when you are at the right school for you.

SEVEN

Places to Go, People to Meet

"Keep your face always toward the sunshine, and shadows will fall behind you."

WALT WHITMAN

We got word from Dr. Palmer that the results were in from him presenting "my case" to the Board and immediately went to see him.

He walked us through my history again and basically his entire presentation. I got the feeling that day that Dr. Palmer wanted to do surgery. At least, that's how he presented it to me. The 50 percent going blind thing was not necessarily affecting him like it was my family. Either way, it didn't matter.

He came to us that day and said if we wanted the surgery, we could have the surgery!

My eyes got wide, "Woah! That's big news," I said.

My mom looked at me and smiled, "Wow... that's amazing."

I'm not sure why we were so skeptical that the Board would say no to it, but we were. I still am convinced that the risk of me losing my eyesight was a bigger deal for my family than it was for the hospital and doctors. Either way, it didn't matter, I was a candidate! Now, we had decisions to make.

"Okay, well, you know I'm leaving to go to Purdue in the Fall, right?" I looked at Dr. Palmer and said.

"Yes. I know."

"If we have this surgery, will I be ready to go by then?"

"Well, this is a major surgery and recovery time will be extensive, so you will probably need to take a semester or two off before you go there."

That was all he needed to say to me. The answer was no. I could not wait to get to Purdue, and that was all that mattered to me at that point in my life. Dr. Palmer did make one major change before college and I'm extremely grateful to him for that now.

Because I only had nocturnal seizures (meaning I only had seizures when I was sleeping), Dr. Palmer had me take most of my medication before bed. His theory was the same as before. He started the process for that when we first started seeing him, but he changed it even more before I left for college. He believed that this would help negate the drowsy feelings that all the other medications were giving me during the day, and I'd sleep off some of the side effects. I'll give him credit on that one for sure. That was one of the best changes a doctor has ever made for me. I could feel a difference when we made that adjustment. It definitely helped me, in my opinion.

I was going to live with epilepsy... for now.

> *Abby's Advice*
>
> Ask about small adjustments that can be made to help with side effects. Seizure medications make me very tired. Dr. Palmer's recommendation to take a higher dosage at night so that I could sleep some of the side effects off made a huge difference for me. Ask your doctors questions about what they've done for other patients having difficulties with side effects.

COLLEGE

I met one of my very best friends at Purdue, Kelley Milloy. She and I were roommates freshman year of college. We both were forced by our parents to live in the only all girls dorm on campus. At that point in time, most colleges had already moved to co-ed dorms, Purdue being one of them. But, they kept one dorm for all girls and one dorm for all boys for people like Kelley and me, whose parents were still old school.

Anyway, I got my letter in the mail that summer that Kelley Milloy from Olney, Maryland would be my roommate. I'll never forget this. My mom and I were sitting in the driveway of our house in the car when I opened my freshman year room assignment.

"Kelley Milloy from Olney, Maryland... Ole-nee? Did I say that right?"

I looked over at my mom, and she had a puzzled look on her face.

"That's weird. My sorority sister married a guy with the last name Milloy on the East coast."

"It can't be the same, that's just too weird," I said.

"Is there a phone number on that paper?"

"Yeah. Should I call her?" I asked.

"Sure."

We were sitting right there in her car in the driveway, and I called Kelley Milloy for the first time ever.

"Hello!"

"Hi. Kelley? This is Abby, I think we are going to be roommates at Purdue."

"Oh! Hey! Cool! How are you?!?"

"I'm good. I'm excited! I have a really, really random question for you," I said.

"Okay?" Kelley sounded very confused.

"Is your mom's maiden name Stottlemyer?"

"Yes," she said, totally freaked out by my question, and I in no way, shape or form blame her.

"Oh. My. God. Your mom and my mom were sorority sisters at Purdue!"

"What?!?! MOM! Oh my god, MOM!! Do you know wait, who is your mom, Chris, okay, Chris what again, Chris Gustus?"

Sue yelled from the background… "Yes. That's my sorority sister!"

"Her daughter, Abby, is my roommate!"

We were all laughing hysterically. What a small world?!?! By pure chance, I was now roommates with my mom's sorority sister's daughter. She would turn out to be one of the best friends and best things that has ever happened to me in my entire life. Now, I call Kelley, my angel. Some things happen by chance, but I believe a higher power put Kelley and me together. I was mentally ready to be 100 percent independent, but I still needed help that I didn't want to accept. Kelley always provided that, no questions asked.

THE DISABILITY RESOURCE CENTER

We traveled up to Purdue a day earlier than when we were able to move into the dorms, because my mom made me go to the Disability Resource Center. At this point in time, I thought of myself as different only when I was at a specific doctor appointment or when I was recovering from a seizure. I sure as heck didn't consider myself somebody living with a "disability." Why would I need to go there? Why would I need any special accommodations?

What I didn't realize is that I already had all kinds of accommodations in high school, I just never knew it. My school was so understanding and my teachers never asked any questions. If I needed another day, my mom and dad called the teacher, and there was never any problem. If I had to stay home for a couple of days from school because I needed to recover from a seizure, they just sent my work home with my brother. All the accommodations that were made seemed so effortless that I barely realized that's what they were. Parkway Central teachers and administrators were so helpful, I never had to think about getting "formal accommodations." Neither did my parents for that matter. We never needed it.

My mom was dragging me (not quite kicking and screaming, but close) to the Disability Resource Center at Purdue the day before Kelley and I would move in together on what was going to be one of the best days of my life, and I was miserable. I just had to suffer through this and everything would be okay.

"We have to go and see what they have available for you in case you have a seizure, Abby."

"I won't have a seizure, let's just go, we don't need this."

"What if you have a seizure and you cannot go to class the next day? What if you have a test the day after you have a seizure?"

"So what if I do? Everything will be fine. I don't need to go to a Resource Center for people with disabilities, Mom. This isn't the kind of disability they are referring to, MOM!"

"Let's just go see what they have to offer. Please. We just have to go see."

"Oh my god, you drive me insane. I cannot believe this."

We walked in the office and were greeted by a receptionist, she looked like a student to me. She smiled and handed us a form to fill out, and said, "Take a seat, we will have a staff member with you shortly."

My mom smiled back, "Thank you."

I was still feeling mad at my mom for having me here in the first place, so I sat down next to her and crossed my arms and stared at the floor while my mom filled out the paperwork.

"Abigail Gustus?"

We both looked up. The staff member looked at us and said, "Come on in!"

We both got up and followed the staff member back to her office. It was an office with a great view of the Mall, which is where my attention stayed almost the whole meeting since I was convinced I didn't need any accommodations. I was just here now to humor my mom.

"How can we help you?" she said as she took her seat behind her desk.

My mom looked over at me and I looked back at her with a face of, what the hell are you looking at me for? This was your idea.

"Well, we wanted to come and get a better understanding of accommodations that Purdue has for people with epilepsy."

"Okay… yes, we have students with epilepsy. We can definitely help you. Help me understand your needs."

"Okay, well Abby has grand mal seizures, some people call them tonic-clonic seizures, in her sleep. The seizures cause her to sleep for anywhere from 24 to 48 hours. My fear is that she will have a seizure on the night before a test and not make the test. In high school, we were able to just work directly with her teachers and she was able to make everything up, but I'm not sure that's how it will work here. I just wanted to understand what, if anything, she needs."

"Good. I'm glad you are here. First off, let me tell you that if you are going to miss any assignments, tests, or classes due to a seizure, the only way the professor can excuse it is if you have a letter from our office. So, you've come to the right place.

All of those accommodations are reasonable asks and we are happy to help you. We just need to get some letters from your doctors, some information about the accommodations you have had to date in high school, and we can get you a letter that you will give to your professors."

"Wait, sorry, what did you say about accommodations she's had already?" my mom asked.

"Well, yes. Don't you already have documentation that these sorts of things have already been done for Abby from her high school?"

"No, we just worked it out with her teachers back at home.

There was nothing formal or in writing."

"Hmmmmm… okay, well that might present us with a bit of a challenge. I'm sure it will be fine. It would be easier if we had that already, but that's not going to affect us helping Abby get what she needs."

My mom relaxed and smiled, "Okay, thank you. So, how does this actually work?"

"Well," the DRC staff member said as she looked at my mom, then to me, "Abby, you will get a letter from us, one for every Professor, at the beginning of the semester. Every semester you will have to come pick them up before classes start. We send the Professors the same letter via E-mail, but we ask that all of our students take the Professor a letter after class on the first day and introduce themselves. This gives the Professors the opportunity to meet you and ask any questions they may have. Also, it gives the two of you an opportunity to figure out how you want to handle a situation if you do happen to have a seizure. For example, does the professor want you to E-mail them? Would they like you to call?

Between the two of you, with this letter, you can come up with a mutually agreeable solution if something were to happen. If not, business as usual."

"Okay…" I felt confused and my mom could tell. She jumped in to help clarify for me.

"So, this just means that if you have a seizure on let's say, the night before a test… you can work with your professor to figure out when you can take it once you've recovered rather than try to take it that day when you aren't 100 percent yet."

I nodded my head… it was starting to make sense now.

"Yes, that's exactly right. Mrs. Gustus, there is some formal

105

information we will need from you to make sure that Abby gets these letters before class starts, but we should be fine. We have enough time. I'm sure your doctor will provide us with a note, yes?"

"Yes. I'll call Dr. Palmer right after we get done here. Can you get me the information of where you would like it sent?"

"No problem. I'll meet you out front."

We gathered our things and headed to the lobby of the DRC. She met us there with contact information for Dr. Palmer, shook our hands, and that was that!

It was official. Just like my mom thought/knew, I did need formal accommodations in college. She was not crazy, like I totally thought she was. We also worked with Parkway Central to get a written note from the principal explaining the informal agreement we had had in place for the past four years.

"See... aren't you glad we came here, Abby. You need that letter or it's considered unexcused, and you could end up with a zero. You don't want that."

"No... I definitely don't want that. You were right."

"Let's go call Dr. Palmer... we need him to hurry up and send this letter!"

Dr. Palmer was a huge help and sent the letter right away, as was my principal from Parkway Central.

Before I knew it, I was passing out letters to every single one of my professors. On a huge campus like Purdue, it actually ended up being a small (very small) blessing in disguise. I always got to know every one of my professors, because I had to physically give them this letter. So, all my professors always knew who I was. When you are in a class of 200 to 300 people, that's important especially if you are at an 89.4 percent or something when it's time to give grades. It was nice to get to know them, that's all I'm saying.

Abby's Advice

Growing up, we lived in an area where we were close with all of the teachers, coaches, counselors, etc. at the high school I attended. Therefore, all of my teachers and counselors just worked with me if I ever had a seizure. I never needed any formal documentation to "prove" anything. It was all good faith and there was an understanding I would get the accommodations I needed.

While I am eternally grateful to Parkway Central for making me feel normal and always helping me when I needed it, not having formal documentation backfired in college. We should have, as a family, gone through the formal steps to get those documents in place in high school. Purdue University wanted the documentation to "prove" I had been getting accommodations, and we had nothing to show for it.

If you do need any sort of help whether it's another day to recover from a seizure, or a longer test time period, get it in writing and document it! The resource centers at universities typically need that in writing. Obviously, we worked through it. But, if we would have had it, the process would have gone much smoother.

MY ANGEL

Meeting Kelley on move in day was awesome! We didn't know each other yet, but when we finally met in person, it felt like I had known her my whole life. On top of that, it was a mini-reunion for my mom and Sue, Kelley's mom.

While I felt like I had known Kelley for years, and we were instant friends, I for some reason never, ever told her about my seizures. Deep down, I knew I should, especially now because we would be permanent residents of the same room, but I couldn't bring myself to tell her. I was still very embarrassed about it.

I had been judged and bullied (not a lot, but just enough) in high school to be scared to talk about it. Now, I have no shame in telling people I have epilepsy, but for some reason, I could not work up the courage to tell Kelley.

I should have known better, though. What do you think happened? Good 'ole mom to the rescue again. During the move, without my knowledge (if I would've known I would've killed her) pulled Kelley aside and told her about my seizures. She gave her some tips on seizure first aid, helped her understand what it would look like if it happened, helped her understand how scary it is to see your first one, gave her information about the postictal phase, and gave her both hers and my dad's phone numbers for when (not if) the first seizure happened.

You know Kelley is an amazing friend and person because she never once asked me about it or treated me differently. I never even knew that she knew I had seizures. I'm so thankful that I only found out about the conversation she had with my mom on move in day *after* I had my first seizure in our dorm room. I would have been so embarrassed and worried our friendship would not be the same. I know that's not true now, but I did have those feelings.

"Abs, you doing okay??"

"Yeah…" I said, because I was super groggy. "Did I have a seizure?"

"Yeah… you had a seizure last night. It's okay… just rest. Do you need anything?"

"No, but thank you," and tears started rolling down my cheeks. I felt like I had just betrayed Kelley, because I never told her. I never even gave her any warning! How could I have been so selfish!

"I'm sorry I didn't tell you I have seizures…" I said as I cried.

"It's okay Abs… don't worry. I'm glad you are okay. It's totally okay," Kelley said as she sat on the side of my bed. "Everything will be okay. You doing okay now?"

"Yeah, I'm really tired."

"Yeah, just sleep. I'm going to go run some errands, just sleep and I'll be back to check on you in a little bit, okay?"

"K… thanks Kelley."

"You're welcome."

Right after she left, I finally had my wits about me to call my mom.

"Kelley saw me have a seizure last night," I sobbed into the phone. "I never told her I have epilepsy. I feel terrible, I can't believe I did…"

"Abby… Abby… Abby!"

"Yeah???"

"Abby, it's okay. Kelley and I had a conversation on the

day you moved in to the dorms. I told her…"

"You did???" I was sniffling, "Why did you do that?"

"Well, because I knew this would happen… Kelley called us last night when it happened. We talked through it. She was calm and helped you, and then, we just told her to let you sleep."

Abby's Advice

Fellow epileptics:

You need to tell the people that you most interact with. I am in no way saying you need to shout it from the rooftop. I'm not saying that I ever introduce myself and say, "Hi. I'm Abby, and I have epilepsy." That's not what I'm saying. But, if it's a person that you will be rooming with or spending a considerable amount of time with, tell them. Have information ready for them.

Seizure first aid is a good place to start.

- Always stay with the person until the seizure is over
- Try to stay calm. It will be scary, but stay calm, it should not last more than two minutes.
- Remove any objects that may cause the person harm out of the way.
- Do not try to stop any of the seizures movements. If a person gets up and tries to walk around, help them to the ground to prevent injury.
- Do NOT put anything in a person's mouth.
- After a tonic-clonic seizure, breathing should resume normally. Ensure the person is breathing normally.
- Reassure the person that they are in a safe location and offer to stay with them until they are ready to go back to normal activity.

SORORITY RUSH

I fell back asleep instantly. My body was exhausted. If there is one thing to be said about college, it's that your schedule is pretty much never the same. It's not your standard 8 to 5 schedule that a job provides, it's erratic. You have a couple classes a day (maybe), then downtime, then often times you could be up late studying, if you didn't take advantage of that downtime. You could make college like an 8 to 5 job and stay on a good schedule, but I didn't. I wanted to enjoy college just like everybody else, so I followed the same schedule as everybody else. Seizures or not, I was going to stay up late studying at the computer labs with friends.

In addition to the school aspect, you have the social aspect. I think, for a person with seizures, that is the hardest part. College is a very social environment. If you wanted to, you could go out with friends every night of the week. At that age, I was determined to not let my seizures hold me back. Having a seizure was not a deterrent for me. My attitude then was, so what?

I wish now (all the time) that I had taken better care of myself in college. That first seizure Kelley saw was one of many because of the lifestyle I led. At Purdue, sorority rush happens the first week before second semester. Kelley and I were both rushing. We were legacy Chi Os, but I was also, through my aunts, a legacy at Kappa and Theta.

Sorority rush is hard. It's hard on the girls that are rushing, and it's hard on the girls already in houses. You don't get much sleep, and you are constantly preparing for the next day. Purdue, at the time, had somewhere around 16 houses. Rushees visit all 16 houses in the first two days, then eight, then five, then three respectively. Every night the rushees rank their favorite houses, and the sororities rank their favorite girls. From there, you are "matched."

The last day of sorority rush, I visited Chi Omega, Kappa Kappa Gamma, and Alpha Phi. I was excited about all of them to be honest. Each house had something different and special to offer. Ultimately, though, Chi Omega (the same house my mom lived in while she was at Purdue) felt right. I pledged Chi O and found out the next night they chose me too. I got a bid from Chi Omega! Obviously, my first (and most important call) was to mom to tell her my exciting news, and what was her first question?

You guessed it!

"What about Kelley?"

"Kelley's a Chi O too! We are staying together!"

"That's great, Abs! I'm so happy for you both! Tell Kelley congrats from us!"

At Purdue you get your bid and that same night is Bid Night. Bid Night is a night when all the Freshman pledges come to the house to meet all the girls already in the house. It's a really fun night. I won't spill all our secrets, but it is a night to remember. I loved Bid Night, and as a pledge, it's a really cool experience.

We had a ton of fun with the girls in the house, but it was really late when we finally got to go to bed. At Purdue in the Chi O house, we all slept in "cold air." It's a big room on the top floor of the house with the windows open year round… even in the winter. Everybody sleeps under heated blankets. It sounds crazy, but it's amazing to sleep there. Every once in a while, I wish I had "cold air" in our house! Anyway, on Bid Night you sleep in your pledge mom's bed for the night.

"Abby, here's where you will sleep," my Pledge Mom said.

"Kelley, here's your bed," her Pledge Mom said. We pretty much stayed together the whole day. Our Pledge Mom's picked us up at the dorms together, we did all of our introductions together. They happened to be super close friends too, so it was cool that the four of us got to be together that day and night.

Luckily, Kelley was just steps away from me.

My pledge mom showed me her bed and I felt a pang in the bottom of my stomach. It was on the top bunk. Shoot, I thought to myself.

I was not about to say a word about it though. And, to be honest, my excitement was too great to think anything else of it. I'll never have a seizure on the top bunk on bid night. That will never happen, I thought to myself!

This story is pretty predictable. Stay up late after a long stressful week of rush… that's a recipe for disaster for a person with epilepsy. After we finally got to bed, in front of all of my brand new sorority sisters (who had no idea what epilepsy even was at the time except for two of them, Heidi Prince and Kelley), I had a seizure, on the top bunk. One of my new sorority sisters had a brother who had epilepsy. He, too, is living a happy, healthy life today, but at the time, he was having struggles as well, and Heidi understood them all too well. It was obvious Heidi had a special place in her heart for me with how caring she would always be when I had a seizure throughout college. She, too, provided incredible support for me.

Once again, I was back where I started. This was another example of a time in my life when I was too scared to tell the people (who would be sleeping next to me) that I was epileptic. I do not know why during this time period of my life it was so hard for me to tell people, but I could not get it out. I always felt like I needed people to get to know me first, then I could tell them and it would be okay… but only after they knew me. If they got to know me and saw that I was "normal" first, then judgment wouldn't be as bad. Or they would be able to get past it and not see me as a person living with a disability… or as somebody living with something they didn't want to be associated with.

My memory from the seizure that night is pretty terrible. I'm honestly glad I don't know that much about it, because I think it would devastate me. I know that it scared many of the girls. Obviously, it woke everyone up. Luckily though, as always, Kelley was there. She was there to make sure I didn't hurt myself. She was there to explain to the rest of the girls what was happening. I can't imagine what would have happened that night if Kelley hadn't have been with me.

The nicest part about being in Chi Omega was that nobody judged me. All of my sorority sisters, whether I scared them to death that night or not, got past it and treated me as an equal. The bullying that I felt in high school was never there. For the first time in my life, these girls treated me with love and respect. And, in addition to that, they would protect me from anybody if I was ever bullied. I love them for that, and I think the fact that all of them found that out about me the very first night they met me, and chose to be my friend without judgment anyway… well, it's just something you can never be thankful enough for.

Abby's Advice

No matter what the circumstances are, do not sleep on the top bunk bed. You could fall and seriously injure yourself. It is just not worth it. If you are in a situation where you are uncomfortable explaining why, nicely let the person know you prefer the bottom bunk. Above all, safety first. Sleeping on the top bunk is not a safe place for those of us with seizures.

EIGHT

A Mind of My Own

"A girl should be two things: who and what she wants."

COCO CHANEL

By the end of my Freshman year of college I was sick of having seizures. I was over the feelings of embarrassment because my friends were so accepting. Now I just felt like my seizures were more of a nuisance than anything.

Little things would bug me. One night I was out at a party with my new sorority sisters and realized I had forgotten to take my medicine. A couple of us walked back to the dorms together, got it, and went back out. But, who wants to leave a party to do that?! Not me.

Without even talking to my parents, I decided that summer that I was going to have the surgery. I wanted epilepsy gone forever. I didn't care about the risks. My mind was made up.

My parents picked me up from Purdue, and we made the trek home. Once we got there, my mom, my dad and I were sitting in our family room having a nice, pleasant conversation about

Purdue. We were talking about all of my new friends, Chi Omega, and my major. I abruptly changed the subject.

"I'm going to have brain surgery this summer. I want to meet with Dr. Palmer. Can we get an appointment?" I said.

"What?" my mom said.

"Yeah. I'm ready for it now. Seizures are too annoying. I don't want to have them anymore."

"Well… there are a lot of risks associated…"

"I don't care anymore… I want these to be gone. I'm sick of having seizures! I don't want to be scared to sleep in the house (referring to the Chi Omega sorority house) and be worried I'm going to scare everyone! I don't want to walk all the way across campus to get medicine late at night because I forgot it! I don't want to have a seizure and worry about my head getting stuck! It's not okay!"

In that instance I was referring to a very, very scary night where Kelley saved my life when I was having a seizure. My head got lodged in between my dresser and my bed when I started my seizure in our dorm room. Somehow it was cutting off my air circulation and had Kelley not been there to reposition me, I would have choked because my body was stuck. So, Kelley literally did save my life in college, not just emotionally, she physically did.

Kelley never told me that story, of course. My mom did (after the fact) when she was trying to explain how important it was that I not get overtired and stressed. That was one of the hardest stories to hear… ever.

So, I was over it. And, Dr. Palmer had the answer.

"We need to talk about this a little more. Your dad and I don't really think the surgery is a good solution," my mom said as she looked at my dad.

"Yeah… that's not happening," my dad said. He always had a way of telling me exactly what I didn't want to hear. It was probably mutual though.

"Why do you get to decide?" I glared at him. "It's not your body. It's not your brain! It's mine!" my voice was escalating quickly.

"We just aren't going to take that risk," he said matter-of-factly and shrugged his shoulders. He was calm. I, on the other hand, was not.

"Why dad? That's so stupid! You don't know what it's like?!? You don't get to make that decision, I do!"

"Actually, *we* get to make it," he said as he pointed one finger to my mom and then back to himself. "Your mother and I do, and the answer is no."

I looked at my mom, this was not what I expected to hear from them. I could have sworn they would be excited that I wanted to have the surgery. Did they expect I was going to change my mind?

It felt to me like they were very prepared for this conversation. They must have known that I might come home with this information, they knew me too well. I knew back then in my heart of hearts, it really wasn't the best idea. But, in college you feel invincible. That's how I felt the summer after Freshman year.

But, surgery was off the table. My dad made that very clear.

Abby's Advice

Brain surgery is a huge risk no matter what the circumstance. Carefully weigh your options before making an impulse decision. Understand all the risks and not just the major ones. You need to know all of them. Have your doctor write them down for you, so you can refer back to them later once emotions have settled.

DEAR BYRON

I spent that summer dreaming of when I could get back to Purdue. I stayed in close contact with my new friends and just wanted to be back. That summer was the last time I'd ever have a seizure at my parent's house.

I was resting that day. It was a weekend, and I was probably out too late the night before. It was the middle of the day, and I laid down to take a nap. I was asleep within minutes.

As I started having more and more seizures (as I did in college), I realized that if I could wake up right before a seizure and focus on something else, sometimes I would be able to stop the seizure from happening. This was rare, but it had happened before. Waking up would make it so I would not have a seizure. It's only worked a couple times in my lifetime. But, what my body started doing was waking me up right before it. It's one of the scariest feelings ever, because 99 percent of the time, there's nothing you can do except have the seizure and let it pass.

I jolted up in bed. My heart was racing. I could feel a

seizure coming on. Shoot! I thought to myself. I instantly got up and walked into the hallway.

"DAD! DAD HELP!!!" I screamed bloody murder.

"I'm going to have a seizure." I started frantically pacing around in circles. Pacing. Pacing. Back and forth. Back and forth.

Instantly, Byron and my dad were upstairs with me.

"I'm going to have a seizure," I was scared looking up at my dad for help.

"Okay… it's okay," my dad said looking at me frightened.

"I'm going…" I collapsed into his arms and had a seizure right there in the middle of the hallway. Byron was there to watch the whole thing.

They must have carried me to bed, because I woke up much later. I walked downstairs after I had recovered just enough to make it downstairs to the family room where my dad was sitting.

"I had a seizure, didn't I?" I said to my dad as I sat down on the couch.

"Yeah… you had a seizure. You okay?" he said and looked at me from across the room.

"Yeah. I'm fine. I bit my tongue, I'm going to need to go get some Orajel."

Orajel is my saving grace after a seizure. Biting your tongue or cheek is so painful. It's hard to eat, hard to talk, it's pretty miserable for at least a few days if it happens..

"I think you need to go talk to Byron," my dad said. "He's been crying."

"Why has he been crying?"

"It's really hard to watch, Abby. He's upset."

"Really?? It upset him that much?"

I never expected my little brother (who was not little anymore, he was going to be a senior in high school) to care. Why did he care?

"Yes, Abby. Go talk to him and let him know you are okay when you're up to it."

"Okay."

I never talked to Byron that day. So, I'm formally apologizing here. Sorry By! Love you! I know, I know. It's not a joke. And, I really am very sorry.

For me, those were the most impactful moments. Seeing my family completely distressed and distraught was way worse for me than the seizure itself. I can deal with the seizures all day. I cannot deal with the people I love the most in pain because of something that happened.

I know they know I can't help it. But, the thing is… I can help it. I can be responsible and make sure I don't get overtired. I can make sure I take my medicine. I can do little things to help myself. That story was like a dagger to my heart. As much as I loved teasing and basically tormenting Byron, I never would do anything to hurt him. And that day, he was hurt. It was not worth it.

Abby's Advice

Fellow epileptics:

As I said before, this disorder affects families. It greatly affects siblings, because often times, the seizures, doctors' visits, caretaking, etc. take so much of your parents energy and time. As a child, that is difficult on your siblings. That's on top of it being absolutely devastating to see someone you love having a grand mal seizure. Just keep that in mind, and give your sibling or siblings a hug, because they have been through a lot, too.

If you have questions, please feel free to E-mail me at seizethedayabby@ gmail.com and I will do my best to answer. If I cannot answer your questions, I will share any relevant resources or try and point you to someone who can.

NINE

Big Cities, Bigger Dreams

"Life is either a daring adventure or nothing at all."

HELEN KELLER

I was back at Purdue before I knew it, and moving into the sorority house. It felt amazing. I was excited to be back with all the girls who provided me so much support when they hardly even knew me. The support that group of girls provided me during such a fragile time in my life is something that will always hold a special place in my heart. And, on top of that, I know my parents are eternally grateful as well.

That said, their acceptance and love gave me the ability to be myself and thrive.

By then, I was seeing possibilities and not just seizures. My major in college was Speech Pathology and Audiology, but by my Junior year, I was getting tired of it. I enjoyed it but couldn't see myself in Speech Path forever. I do feel like those classes, outside of Phonetics (that was hard for me), never challenged me as much as I would have liked. I think a lot of it had to do with the fact that

I spent so much time growing up at my mom's school and working with children who are deaf or hard-of-hearing.

I spent my summers as a teacher's aide at the Moog Center for Deaf Education, where my mom works. I was a teacher's aide and helping teach kids sophomore, junior, and senior year of high school during the summer. Either way, I had a lot of experience with what we were studying in those classes and felt bored. I started taking Communications and Marketing classes as a way to change up my schedule a little bit and fell in love.

My new goal was to be a Journalist, and nobody was going to stop me. I wanted to be a Journalist more than anything. I went and got a job at The Exponent, Purdue's student newspaper Freshman year. I was in love! This was where I belonged. I started as a staff writer and by Sophomore year, I was the Campus Editor.

I loved writing stories about the goings on on campus. My friends loved me writing stories too, because I could always use them as sources and publish their names as the "student quotes" or use their names when I would do a "from the student's perspective" piece.

I know that's against every rule in the journalism book (to use sources you know) but it was college and we were having fun with it. The most exciting story I ever covered was when a car drove through the front door of our local soda shop called The Den. Believe me, that was big news at the time!

I thrived at the Exponent and started to believe a career in Journalism was where I wanted to be. I needed some experience... fast. That led to my first big internship the summer after my Junior year in college.

THE ABRAMS REPORT

I am a self-proclaimed news junkie, and I think that's how I ended up at The Exponent one day looking for a job. I wanted more though. I wanted to know what it would be like to work at a major network. The summer before my junior year when I was working for my grandpa, Buddy, I sent resumes and cover letters to every major news source I could think of. I sent letters to 20/20, MSNBC, CNN, Nightline, Dateline, The TODAY Show, Good Morning America, literally, all of them. Luckily, I worked for my grandpa, and he was very understanding about me spending at least half my time "working" on cover letters and resumes.

I was determined.

I'm sure you've all heard the saying, all it takes is one. Well, that's true. One day, I got a phone call from MSNBC and they wanted to interview me right then and there on the spot via phone. Jodi, who ran the internship program for MSNBC and who I am still grateful to today, asked me questions about my background, my interests, what my career goals were, and more. I answered all her questions as best I could with no preparation time.

Finally, at the end of the conversation, I asked, "Would it be helpful if I just came up there to meet you for an hour or two?"

I could've never imagined her answer to be, "Yes! When can you be here?"

It was a whirlwind, but within a couple days my mom and I were on our way to New York City. The MSNBC

Headquarters was in Seacaucus, N.J. just across the river when we went to visit. I'll never forget that day. I told Jodi ahead of time that my mom would be coming with me to New York City since it was my first time. She immediately said, bring her with you to the studio, and I'll give you both the tour.

I'm not sure who was more excited about that tour. My mom or me… I think, ultimately, my mom took the cake.

Jodi never formally sat me down and interviewed me in the traditional sense. We talked as we walked around the studio. She showed me where all the different teams for each show sat. At the time, there were teams for Hardball with Chris Matthews, Countdown with Keith Olbermann, The Abrams Report with Dan Abrams, and more, but those were the most prominent at the time. It was really cool to see. After that, she asked us if we wanted to see the actual studio where the teams were on air.

I think both of our eyes lit up like it was Christmas morning.

"Okay, I'll take that as a yes," she said.

"Yes. Yes. Please."

We quietly stepped out onto the studio floor and right in front of our eyes, Lester Holt, who is now the anchor on Nightly News, was doing his mid-day broadcast.

Now, this sounds cheesy, but I actually played it pretty cool. After all, this was an interview. But, oh my goodness… my mom lost it.

I looked at her and said, "Mom, please try to be cool." I gave her… the look.

"But, Abby, that's Lester Holt. I watch him ALL. THE. TIME."

She played it just cool enough for us to walk out of the

studio without her begging him for an autograph right then and there in the middle of his live broadcast.

We got back to where we started at the front door, and Jodi asked, "Which show do you see yourself interning for?"

"I'm not really sure. Maybe Hardball?"

To be completely honest, that was the only show that I really knew about at the time. I had never heard of the other news shows. I was not yet focused on national and international news. At Purdue, I had a tough time getting out from behind West Lafayette campus news, so I was a little unprepared for that question.

"Well, can I be honest... with everything you've told me and from our conversations, I really see you fitting in best on The Abrams Report with Dan Abrams and the team there. That show focuses more on legal, crime, and tabloid issues," Jodi said.

I couldn't hide my excitement, "Yes. That's *exactly* the kind of show I want to work on!"

"So, you are in?"

"Yes!"

It was so cool, I walked out of the studio that day (with my mom, which was a little funny, but I was still in college) with my first real summer internship. There was one minor issue, where would I live and with who?

Fate works in mysterious ways, because that problem was solved rather quickly. That summer, one of my closest friends from high school, Laura Korbecki, also had an internship in New York City. Her internship was with MetLife. Laura was going to Indiana University, so I actually did see her on a regular basis when our two schools would play each other in football or there happened to be just another fun party to attend because we were so close.

Most importantly, Laura knew me from high school and was well aware that I had epilepsy. I did not have to stress about telling her or worry what she would think. She knew. She was one of a few friends who visited me when I had my Video EEG at Children's.

So, to say the least, it worked out! We roomed together at the New Yorker hotel, just a couple blocks away from Time Square. How amazing is that?!?

Our room that summer was pathetically small. Looking back on it, I'm not even sure how we lived there. Our furniture consisted of two twin beds with desks and chairs. The desks were back to back in the middle of our beds, and there was not enough room for the chairs! We had to sit on our bed to work at our desks. We had no kitchen and only one half size closet. Our bathroom was super small, but luckily we had to be at work at different times. That is the only way getting ready in the morning was possible.

It was such a fun summer. She and I did everything possible super tourist-y. We visited every single "local" attraction New York had to offer. We had a cameo on the Today Show at the John Legend concert as well! It was fantastic!

What I took away from that summer was that a set schedule really agreed with me. I only had one seizure the summer that I lived with Laura. That was a really good stretch for me in my college days. It also happened early on a Saturday morning, so I recovered and never had to miss a day of my internship! Thank goodness! It was the first time in three years that I was not up late on random occasions and every day had a set schedule. It helped... a lot.

Laura was calm and collected the early morning that it happened. We had openly discussed what could happen if I did have a seizure. By that time, I was more confident in talking about it, so I think that helped to ease any nerves she may have had as well.

That summer in New York City and the internship that I had solidified my love of journalism and television news. It was the summer of the Michael Jackson trial and the Natalee Holloway disappearance in Aruba. There were more, but those were the two stories that dominated the news cycle that summer. There were new updates every day, and we reported all of them. I loved it!

The newsroom erupted the day Michael Jackson was found innocent of the sexual abuse charges. I remember it being chaotic. People were screaming, "There's a verdict!"

I still get excited when breaking news happens, and I am glued to the TV. I am so thankful that I had that opportunity. I got to work alongside some of the most famous newscasters in the business and work with one, in particular, daily.

Dan Abrams was kind enough to write me a letter of recommendation once I decided I wanted to go to graduate school for Journalism. I think his letter (that he actually made me write so he could sign it... that was my first real taste of corporate America) was what helped me. I put in way more effort to getting into graduate school than I ever put into getting into undergrad. I could tell I cared... a lot.

I applied to six Journalism schools all over the country and got accepted to two.

ACCEPTED

I'll never forget the day I got my acceptance letter from

Northwestern. It came while I was living with my sorority sisters senior year in what we called "the apartments." We had an entire block of apartments, four girls to an apartment. I opened up the letter and read it. I was shaking (in a good way people)! I read it over and over. Nobody at my apartment was home at the time, so I ran next door.

"Kozon! Read this… read this to me. Does this mean I got in?" I asked her, sounding completely frantic.

"Hang on… let me read it," Laura said (we called her Kozon, and we still do today, even though she's married… her last name now is Atkinson).

I looked at her, eyes wide open as she read through the letter carefully.

"Yes. You got in!"

I was so excited! The letter read a little weird because they wanted me to start a quarter later than I had originally planned. I honestly could not tell if it was an acceptance letter or not.

We hugged.

"Yay Abs! I'm so proud of you!"

"Thank you! I cannot even believe it! It does not feel real!"

I love Kozon for that special moment she shared with me that day.

Of course, the next call was to my parents. They were just as excited!

"Ace!!! Abs got in to Northwestern!"

"Oh. My. God," said my dad.

I knew my parents were ecstatic for me. They understood how badly I wanted to go to graduate school. What a day that was! Before I knew it, I was graduating from Purdue University with two degrees, because I waited so long to make up my mind about what I actually wanted to do. I had a Bachelor of Science in Speech Pathology and a Bachelor of Arts in Mass Communication. I was proud of both.

I look back on college as one of the most special times of my life. I see a time when I had a lot of seizures... too many to count. I am mad at myself for letting that happen, but again, I hadn't hit my tipping point yet. And when I say that, I mean that I still needed to hit that point of I've had enough. Everybody around me had gotten there, but I still hadn't. Nobody else wanted me to have seizures. But, for some reason, I just was not there. I didn't want to have them, that was obvious when I wanted the surgery. But, I wanted a quick and easy fix. I did not want to focus on taking care of my body and changing my lifestyle to accommodate epilepsy.

I think when you are young, some of the negative effects that seizures are having on your body are hard to recognize. The most hurtful thing I have to deal with now as an adult is my terrible memory. There are huge gaps in my memory. For example, people will ask, "Do you remember when we did such and such with so and so?" or "Remember that time..." I'll have absolutely no clue what they are talking about. Friends and family will be sitting there reminiscing and everyone will be talking about something we did or the things we saw, and I'll have nothing to offer to the conversation. It is literally a blank slate for me. It's as if somebody went into my brain and erased the entire encounter from my memory. Sometimes even entire trips that we took as a family are gone from my memory.

My adult self wants to go back in time and tell my younger, invincible self that this will all catch up to you. With every seizure you have, yet another precious memory could be erased... forever.

THE NEXT STEPS

Not long after I graduated from Purdue, I was in Chicago searching for an apartment. It was exciting and scary all at the same time.

Chicago was the first place I'd live, ever, alone... 100 percent independent and by myself. I found a great studio apartment in Lakeview, just outside Lincoln Park in Chicago (it was all I could afford in the City), but I loved it.

When Laura and I lived in New York City, our room was not even big enough for us to have chairs at our desks that were back to back in the middle of our room, so this place seemed spacious!

I was excited about Northwestern's graduate school program, because it was like a job. We had class every day (like a real 8 to 5 job) for one year. Most grad school programs were two to three years, but Northwestern's program was set up for one full year... four quarters. One year in one of the most prestigious journalism schools in the country, and I would be the next Katie Couric. I'm just kidding. Luckily, by then, I was dead set on being a producer behind the scenes. I learned from The Abrams Report that I loved being in the control room. To be honest, almost all the decisions of what goes on the air and what is reported are made by producers behind the scenes, not the on-air team.

That interested me far more.

Grad school was eye opening and taught me a lot. I figured out while I was at Northwestern a couple things. One, I had no interest in local news and that's most likely where I was going to have to start unless I was ready to move right back to NYC… which I was not. And two, I needed more money to live than what a local news network or an Assistant Producer (if I was lucky) in NYC would pay. My grand plan was falling apart at the seams.

My mom and dad told me over and over that I probably would need to change up my lifestyle, financially that is, if I wanted to be a journalist. I never believed them until I was at Northwestern and exposed to the not so glamorous side of the business… something I desperately needed to see. Working at MSNBC was one of the best experiences of my life, but it was not a realistic view of what a first year, right out of school, journalist would be doing. I'd be covering local news not national news. At Northwestern, we would only cover local news. If I was not even interested in covering news for one of the largest cities in America, there was a good chance that a small market was not going to meet my needs. I knew that.

I needed other options… and fast.

Luckily for me, Northwestern also had an absolutely amazing business school and as students of the Medill School of Journalism, you are allowed to take classes there. That's exactly what I did. Every chance I got, I was over at the Kellogg School of Business taking another MBA course.

I'm sure you can imagine by this time, school was hard. The numerous seizures that I'd had throughout high school and college made things that were never difficult for me before, really hard. For example, word finding became difficult for me. It started to show when I would have to write stories quickly and efficiently. I would often get around it and use other words, but it was becoming more and more apparent. Problems I never had noticed before were popping up in my young adult, semi-grown up life.

Grad school was really hard with these small little inconveniences starting to make their way into my everyday life. At the same time, it was really fun, and those inconveniences were just that. I spent all day, every day, with my friend Jackie (Jacqueline Ingles if you live in Tampa and watch ABC News). When we had class in Evanston, we would take turns driving north from the city to campus. When we had class downtown, we would meet at the Belmont Brown Line 'L' stop and take the train to the State/Lake stop.

Jackie and I met the very first night of orientation and were instant friends for life. She went on and pursued the journalism gig, so I still always live vicariously through her. She just won an Emmy last year, and yes, I can brag about her a little, because I'm so proud of her!

While Jackie went on to pursue her career in journalism, I was clueless on where to start. I had come to the conclusion that a career in journalism probably was not for me, yet I could not quite put my finger on what would be a good fit. I knew I really enjoyed the business classes that I was lucky enough to have the opportunity to take, and I loved the marketing classes offered even more. Maybe that was where I needed to focus my attention.

ON-AIR

I did start focusing all of my efforts on business and marketing classes, but I was still required to take all of my J-school classes. After all, my master's was in Journalism. At the time, Northwestern's graduate students had a weekly news program on the PBS channel. We all rotated anchoring the show. It was a big deal to be the anchor. Obviously, that was on-air time in a huge market. Granted, it was on PBS, but that did not matter. It was a big deal, and it was finally my turn to anchor. I had to be up in Evanston, in full hair and make-up, around noon.

The thought of having to be on-air had me completely stressed out. Being stressed is one of my top triggers, just behind missing a dose of medicine and lack of sleep. It's up there. Needless to say, I was extremely nervous about it. The thought of being on-air at the anchor desk the next day had me anxious and terrified.

I remember looking at the clock that night thinking, if I go to bed now, I will get eight hours of sleep. If I go to bed now, I will get seven hours of sleep... and so on. Once I finally got to sleep from pure exhaustion, I had a seizure. All that stress triggered a grand mal seizure.

I was living alone at the time, so nobody was there to confirm it and say yes, you had a seizure last night, but I knew. I always know. My alarm went off around 7 A.M. and I woke up groggy and confused. I stumbled into the bathroom hunched over knowing that I probably had just had a seizure. I looked at myself in the mirror. My hair was a tangled mess. My eyes were swollen and looked like hell. I stuck out my tongue to examine the damage. Yep. It confirmed everything I already knew. During the seizure, I had gnawed the entire right side of my tongue. Teeth marks lined the side of my tongue.

Damn it! I thought to myself. What was I going to do?! I needed to sleep first. I knew in the back of my mind I had about three hours to lay back down and try to semi-recover. Under normal circumstances, I would have taken at least a day, maybe even two. But, this time, I did not have that luxury. My grade depended on this. Yes, I had all the necessary accommodations and technically, nothing could have happened to me, but that was not the point. This was mandatory, and I was going to make it.

I called Jackie to give her the news and let her know I needed a little more time today.

"Oh, Abby, are you okay? What do you need? How can I help?" she asked.

"I just need to sleep for a few hours and when you pick me up I need to stop and get some Orajel for my tongue."

"Okay… okay… no problem."

"Can you also call me at 10 A.M. to make sure I'm awake and getting ready? I cannot miss today."

Jackie understood. She did not try to convince me to just stay in bed. We all knew the importance of this day for our program. You *had* to be there that day.

"Yeah… I know, I understand. I'll call you. If you need anything before then, call me right away."

"Okay. Thanks," I said as I got back in bed and hung up. I laid back down and rolled over to my nightstand where I always kept a glass of water and my medicine. I took two doses for good measure and drifted off to sleep.

My phone rang promptly at 10. Jackie was on it for me.

"Hey… how are you? Can you get up?"

"Yeah… I think I'm going to be okay. I'm going to take a shower and call you back."

"Okay. Let me know."

"Okay. Bye."

Once again, I stumbled back into the bathroom. I was

alright, but my body felt like I had just run a marathon. Every limb felt like it had a fifty pound weight hanging on it. I was going to power through. My mind was made up.

I showered. It was exhausting. Every single thing I did that day winded me. Drying my hair was a victory in itself.

I went back to my bed and sat down for a second before getting dressed. I leaned over and rested my hands on my knees. I was out of breath. I rallied and went into my closet to find my black suit. Luckily, I had been through what I was going to wear on the day I was anchoring a million times in my mind already. I don't think I would have had the energy to pick something out that day.

I got dressed and started doing my makeup. My hands tremored. I put on base, bronzer, and blush, and decided that was as good as it was going to get today. Eye makeup was the most important part of going on-air, but there was no way I was going to be able to put it on that day. We'd had tutorials from teachers about eye makeup, because it was *that* important. But, not to me that day. The basics were good enough.

I called Jackie back to let her know I was ready to be picked up. At that point, we were running a little behind, so I went ahead and called my professor, Beth. I gave her the heads up of what had happened. I let her know Jackie was with me and that we would be there shortly. She told me that I could stay home, but she also knew the importance of this day and did not force the issue.

I looked one last time in the mirror. I looked like I had been hit by a bus. My eyes were swollen and tired. My face was flushed, not in a good way. But, I had to keep moving. I downed one more dose of medicine for another good measure, gathered my laptop and school bag, and headed downstairs to meet Jackie.

She pulled up and got out of the car to give me a hug.

"I'm okay," I said as tears welled up in my eyes.

"I'm so sorry, Abby," she said as she hugged me. "Here, let me get your bags. Where do we need to stop?"

"Walgreens," I said.

"No problem… get in and we will go there first."

"Okay… thank you."

I felt like I was in a cloud… drifting along. This was not the way my first on-air experience was supposed to go. I was supposed to be alert and looking my best. Today, I felt like a second rate version of myself. Ugh…

I got out and went into Walgreens to grab some Orajel. Orajel is a numbing gel that you can put in your mouth. Typically, it's used for babies who are teething or for people who are having tooth aches. It definitely was not designed to numb somebody's tongue after a seizure, but that's what I used it for.

"I can tell your tongue hurts from the way you're talking," Jackie said when I got back in the car.

"You can? Shoot!"

"No, it's not bad… it's just because we are best friends. I just know it's bothering you."

"Yeah… it hurts really bad," I said as I pulled down the visor to open the mirror once again and assess the damage.
"Ugh… this looks bad," I said as I put Orajel on my tongue.

I hate the taste of Orajel. It makes me sick. I think it's mostly mental. It does not actually taste bad, but because of what I have to use it for… it makes me physically nauseous to think about Orajel. Either way, that day, it was a lifesaver. Thank goodness for Orajel.

We pulled into school and had a hike over to the studio. I

thought to myself… you just have to get there then you can take a break. You can sit down for a while once you get there. The walk was not any longer than normal, but that day it felt like our building was miles away. Jackie helped carry my bag. She knew I was exhausted.

We walked in and the whole class was already gathered and ready to go. Every person had "assignments" on the day the show taped. Jackie was in the control room the day that I was on-air. She'd be acting as the producer of the show.

We got there just in time and literally had no time to prepare or anything. It was go time.

I stepped up into the anchor chair and took a seat next to my male classmate, who would be my co-anchor for the show. This is not how I dreamed this special moment would go. Even though I had no dreams of being an anchor, this was a unique and cool experience. I should have been enjoying the moment. It was the total opposite.

The lights went on, and the show started!

I was reading the teleprompter and having a pretty hard time. First, reading a teleprompter is harder than it looks when you haven't had a seizure the night before. Factor that in, yikes. It was really tough.

I'll never forget this. I made a huge mistake on-air. Huge. I read the teleprompter wrong and made a face at the camera. Whatever you do in television, you do *not* do that. Beth stopped the whole show. In my ear piece I heard, "Because of the circumstances, I'm not going to yell at you, but Abby, that was bad. Don't do that again."

My heart sank. She was right. I cannot believe I did that.

It was a low point. I was so upset. I felt like crying but held my composure and finished the show. Everybody knew the mistake I made was huge, but not everybody knew what I had been through physically... just Beth and Jackie. But, still...

That day sucked. Really, really bad. The show aired, and to be honest, other than the fact that I had no eye makeup on, you probably wouldn't have been able to tell anything was truly wrong. But, it was. That day was trying. It was definitely one of the harder days I've ever had... mostly, because I could not take the time I needed to recover. That day taught me a very hard lesson, though.

I know now that I need to take the time I need to recover. Making a huge mistake, because I am tired and not thinking clearly is just not worth it. Not worth it at all.

THE REAL WORLD

The year 2007 was a difficult time for graduates. We were in what history would later refer to as a recession, and from my perspective, nobody was hiring. My lease was about to be up in Chicago. I was about to graduate with a Master of Science in Journalism, and I had no job prospects... zero. The dark cloud of not having a job was getting bigger and life was feeling depressing.

I had the standard call home to mom and dad breakdown, "What am I going to do with my life? I'm never going to find a job! I don't want to move home!"

I started getting desperate. Every interview I went on, I got the same response. You're really qualified, but we just aren't hiring right now. Or, I'd hear, we need a person like you, but you need to have some experience first. How the heck was I supposed to get experience if nobody would even give me a chance?!?

My parents must have sensed my desperation, because my dad sent me a list of the top companies in St. Louis where he thought I should send a resume.

"These are great companies. Even if they don't have an opening that looks interesting to you, just send them your resume," he said.

I had resorted to the fact that I could no longer afford to live in Chicago without a job. I knew I was off the Gustus payroll the day I graduated, so I followed my dad's lead and started applying to those companies. I have no idea why he would send me a construction company, but he did. And, guess what? They had an opening!

The construction company, McCarthy, had a marketing coordinator position in their Healthcare Division open in St. Louis. I was on the health beat at Northwestern, so all my stories during graduate school were health related. That was the same, right?!? Plus, I took business and marketing classes. That was also totally relevant, right?!?

I went in for an interview and with a little luck, and a really amazing manager who was willing to take a chance on me, I had a job! If you would have told me during college or grad school that I would end up at a construction company, I would have told you that you were crazy. But, it's true. I did. My official title was Marketing Coordinator of the Central Healthcare Division. Fancy, huh?!

Real life was staring my adult-self right in the face. It was time for me to get on board too.

FULL CIRCLE

McCarthy needed me to start right away, so I moved back to St. Louis the day classes ended. I was adamant about not moving back in with my parents, so they fronted me the rent money for a two bedroom apartment in Brentwood Forest until I got my first paycheck.

You get a little more square footage for your money in St. Louis. That part was really nice! I moved away from my Chicago friends, but quickly reconnected with one of my friends from high school, Leia Dixon. Leia only lived one street away from me in my new neighborhood. She lived on Canary Cove, and I lived on East Swan. Later, my cousin, Ben, and my brother would move into the same neighborhood as well. Ben lived on Bluebird Terrace and Byron lived on West Swan. See a street pattern there? We had a really great time when we all lived there together. It was short lived, but I loved that time in my life.

Leia and I grew up playing sports together and had known each other since we were in elementary school. Her dad was our basketball coach when we were little. We, unfortunately, were pretty terrible, and I think the score of our games was somewhere in the ballpark of four to two, as in six points were scored total… the entire game.

Needless to say, we had always been friends. As soon as I moved back into Brentwood Forest, though, we became inseparable. We spent all our extra time in the summers at the pool, both the neighborhood pool and the pool at her parent's house. We rotated. Leia and I went to Cardinal games, Blues games, and concerts.

Anytime we could score free tickets from somebody that didn't feel like going that night, we went. We never needed any notice!

Life was good. Work was fun. I loved the people at McCarthy, so I actually really enjoyed my job. And, I lived one street away from my one of my best friends.

I'll never forget the day I got my first bonus check! I had no idea companies even gave those, so it was a huge surprise. I called my dad first, "Wow! Can I have a loan?" he said.

I seriously think he was waiting for that day my entire life… for me to call him and not ask for money.

But, the best part of getting that bonus was the fact that Leia and I had really been wanting a Wii so that we could play Rock Band at one of our apartments. That game was huge back then, and we loved playing with all our friends. We both just didn't really want to splurge on something like that at the time.

So, my next call was to Leia!

"Leia, I just got a bonus! We are going to buy a Wii so we can play Rock Band whenever we want!"

I did not even go home that day, I picked her up and we went straight to Best Buy to get the Wii, the games, the "band" equipment… we got it all! And, yes, skeptics out there, I invested some of it… only some though. I was still only 24 years old. Priorities are a little different at that age. We were young and carefree and had just enough money to have a really good time. So, guess what? We did.

Leia was one of the first friends I had where I was never scared to talk to about my epilepsy. It's ironic, too, because out of all the trips we've taken together and the countless sleepovers we've had, she has never once seen me have a seizure. I think it speaks to the fact that this was a time in my life when I was ready to start taking care of myself.

We went out (a lot), but we also took good care of ourselves. We were both very into health and fitness and still are to this day. One day, I asked Leia if she wanted to try running the GO! St. Louis Half Marathon with me. I was half kidding when I asked her, but she said yes! So, that was that! Leia and I signed up and started training to race.

I had no idea at the time, but running would turn out to be one of my new passions. We both enjoyed it. That race was the first of three we would run together. Moving back to St. Louis and working full time was a great change of pace for me… and for my epilepsy. I could control my schedule and my health, and in turn, I could (for the most part) control my seizures. My health definitely started to take a turn, and finally, it was for the better.

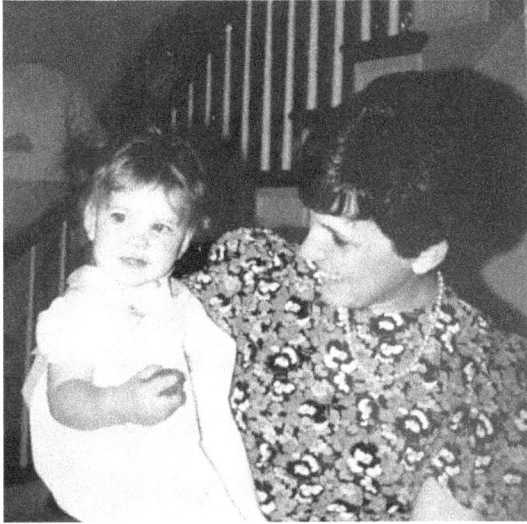

This is one of my favorite pictures of my mom and me. It was taken in St. Louis at a family party. Her smile has and always will be infectious.

Where I was happiest as a kid… at the Lake of the Ozarks. Here I am with my dad and my brother, Byron.

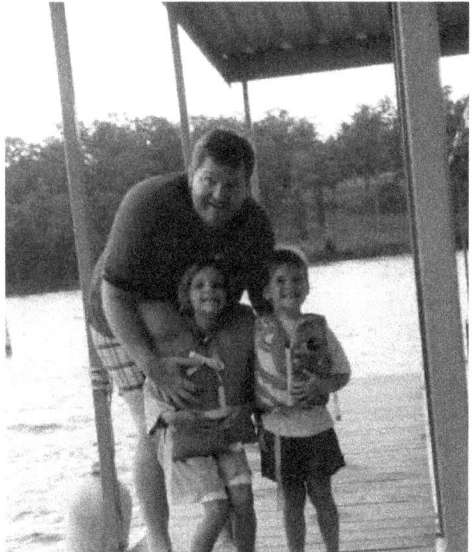

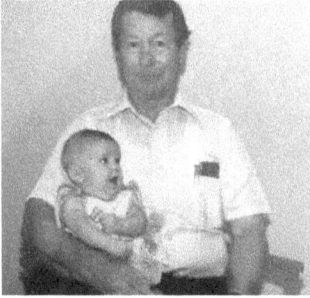

My grandpa, Pop-pop. As I was growing up, he taught me how to drive and play golf… two skills that have always come in handy.

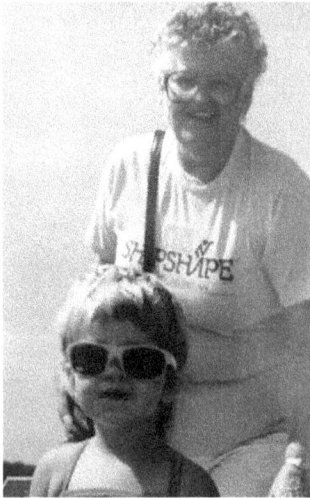

My dad's mom and my grandma, Granny. Here we are at the lake. She was happiest there, too.

Grandma Fran and me at Christmas when I refused to wear anything but dresses and skirts despite the freezing temperatures. She's beautiful inside and out. I learned from her that it is what's on the inside that counts.

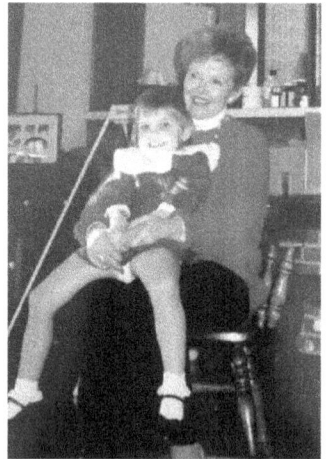

My grandpa, Buddy, who I would later work for, my mom and me on a family trip to California. He taught me all about business and work ethic. My love of reading is also compliments of him.

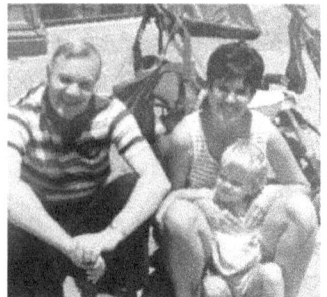

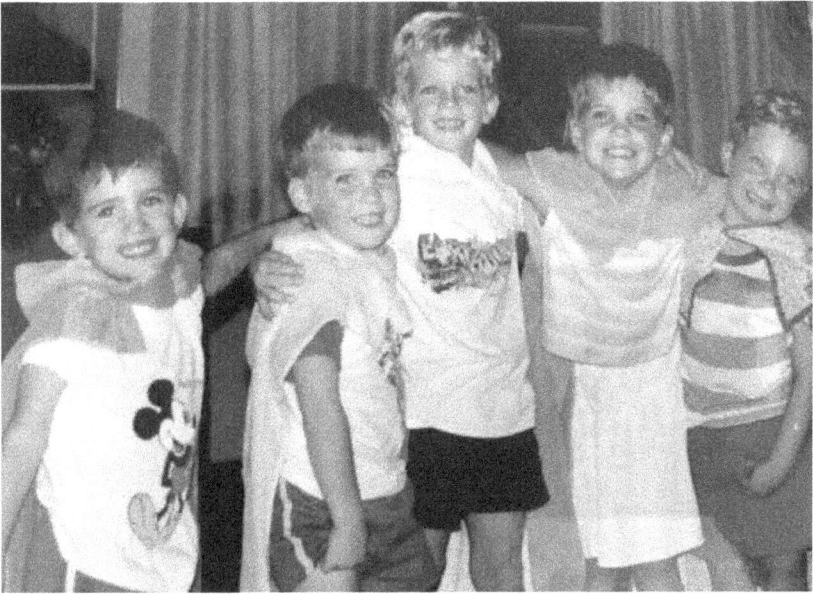

The cousins... We always pinned towels to our backs and played "superman" at Grandma Fran and Buddy's house. That is what you get when you are the only girl in the group. *From left to right:* Danny, Byron, Ben, me, and Matt. I love them all like brothers.

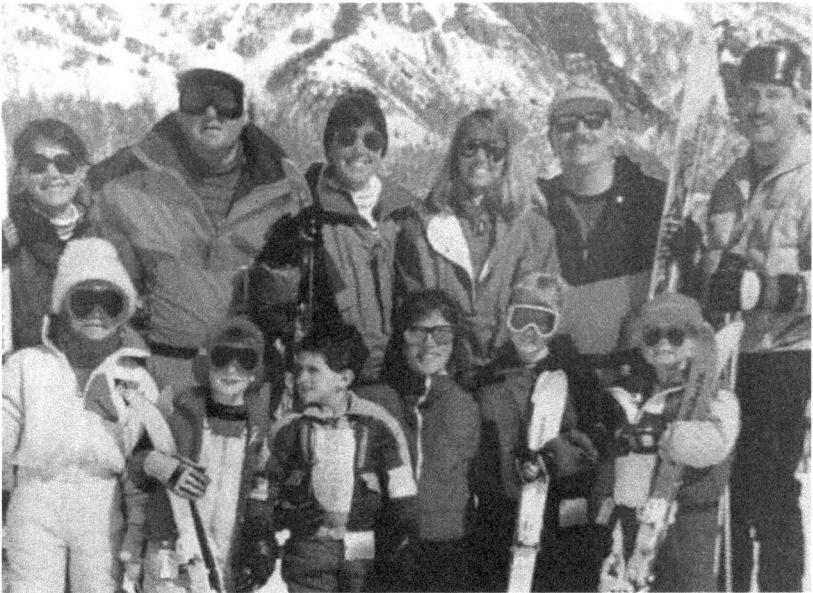

The whole crew! The Hilleary side (my mom's side) went to Keystone in Colorado for a ski trip. This was where Byron and I learned to ski.

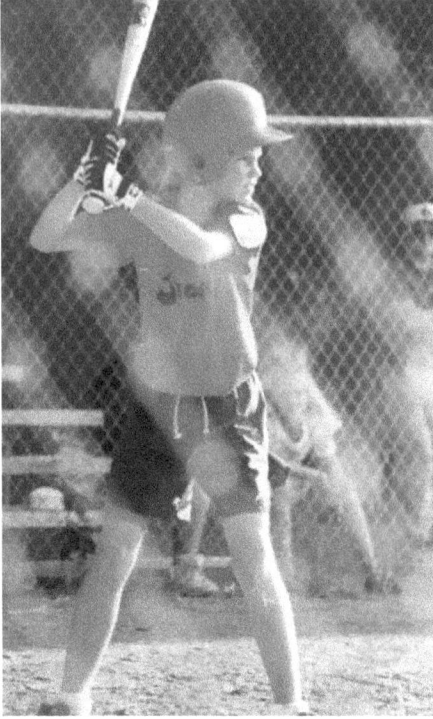

Softball was life for so long. This was the team I played for when I had my very first seizure at the out of town tournament… the St. Louis Storm.

Byron and I on the first day of school. I always loved the first day of school. Byron was starting his freshman year, and I was starting my junior year at Parkway Central High in this picture.

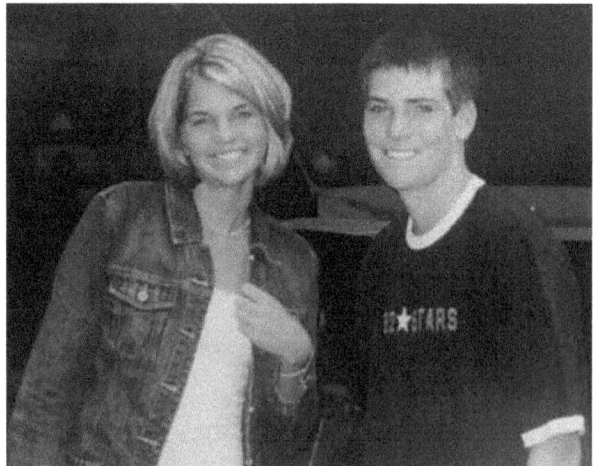

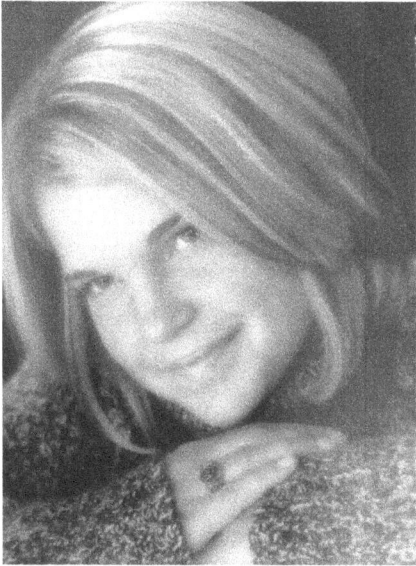

This is my senior picture taken in 2001. I was student council president of our senior class and spoke at our graduation in 2002. It was a very special year for me. I started to see more of what I *could* do rather than what I *could not* do.

Even though I am a terrible singer, I got involved in choir senior year of high school in addition to Student Council. Here I am posing with Byron at a big concert/play we put on called The Madrigal.

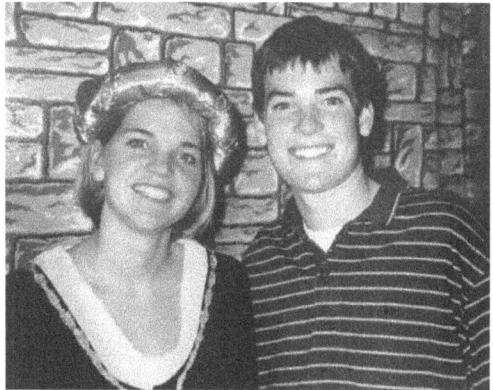

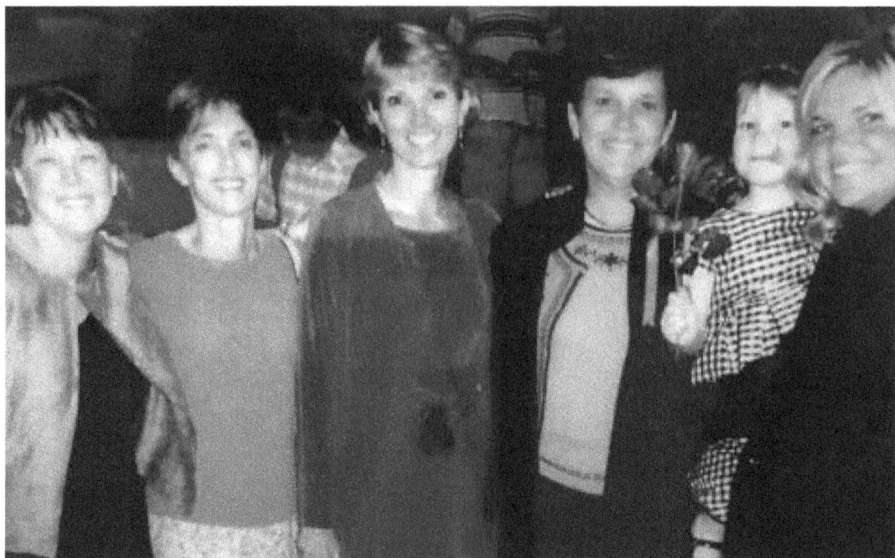

My favorite people, my aunts (my mom's sisters) and my cousin, Holly, who was born when I was 15.
From left to right: Anne, Joan, Nancy, my mom, Holly, and me. I love my boy cousins to death, but I could not wait to finally have a girl cousin after all those years! This was taken at my cousin's high school graduation in La Canada, California.

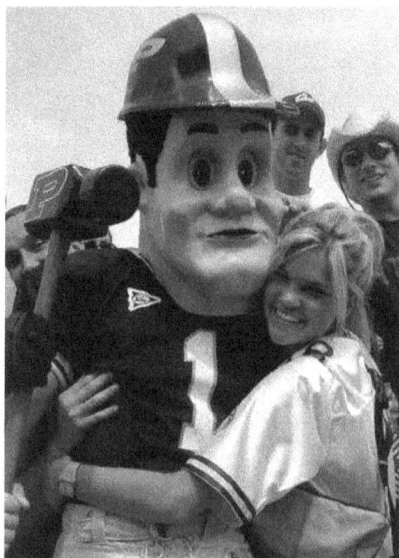

Purdue was (and still is) one of my favorite places on earth. This is a picture of me with Purdue Pete, one of the Boilermaker mascots. Boiler Up!

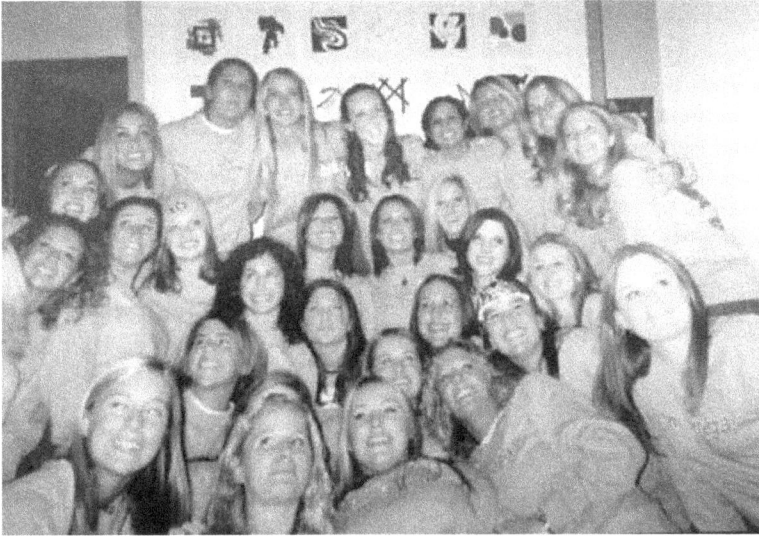

Chi Omega Bid Night. This is the first night I met all of my sorority sisters at the Chi Omega house. Kelley and I are in the top right hand corner of the picture. This was also the night that I had a seizure in front of everyone while sleeping on the top bunk. Thank goodness Kelley was with me.

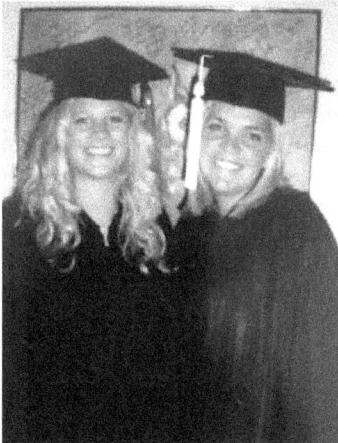

Here I am with Kelley in our cap and gown on graduation weekend. We forgot to take it at graduation so we got all dressed up again to snap one together!

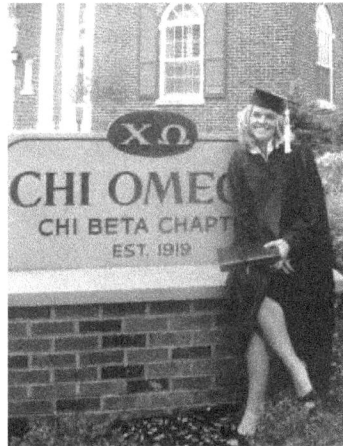

After receiving my diplomas, my family and I stopped by the Chi O house one last time to get a picture.

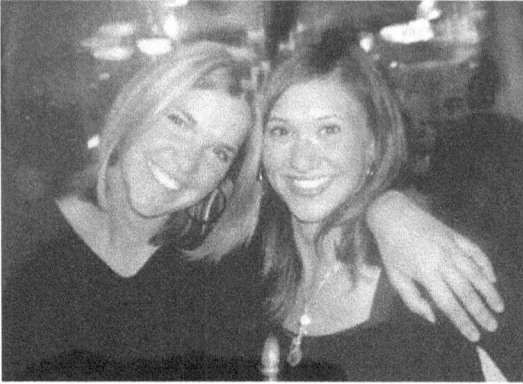

I was lucky enough to meet Jackie on the very first night at Northwestern at our student orientation. We had no idea that night how good of friends we would become.

It was pure coincidence that my friend from high school, Laura, and I would be interning in New York City at the same time. We had a blast that summer together! Here we are a few years later in Minneapolis, where Laura moved for work after college. I went to visit her and we snapped this picture when we were out to dinner.

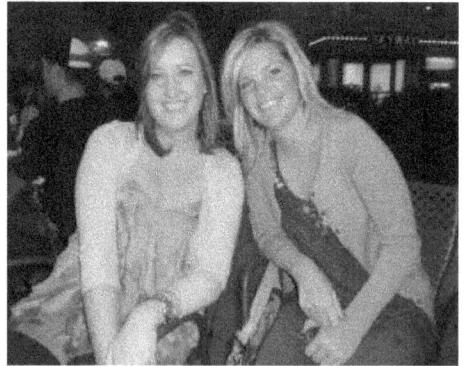

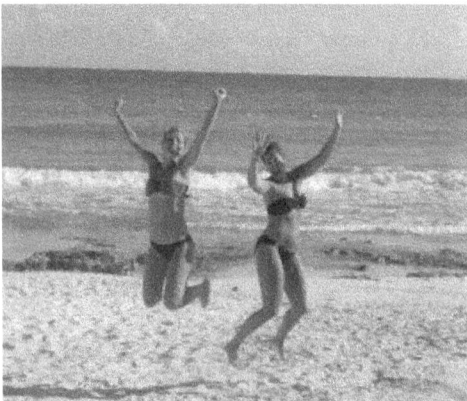

Leia and I have been on many trips together since reuniting in St. Louis in 2007. This was us on vacation with her family doing a beach "photo shoot" in Riviera Maya.

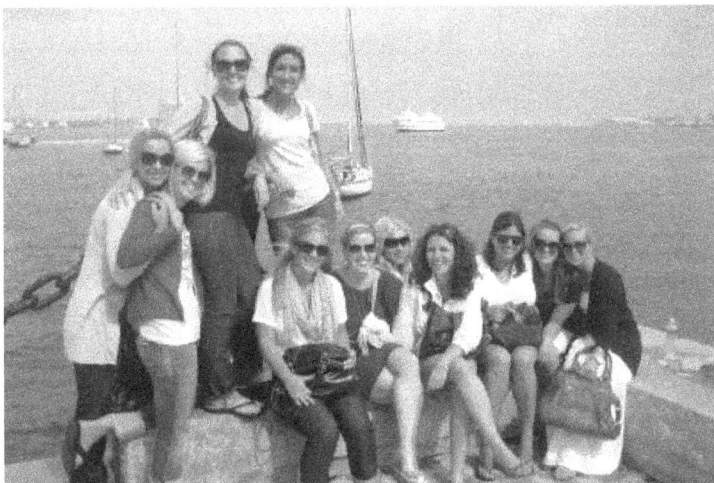

A Chi Omega reunion trip to Boston in 2009. We all met in Boston to visit Kozon, who is now Laura Atkinson.
Back row from left to right: Johnna Perko, me, Danielle (DePotter) Young, Heather Hutton
Front row sitting down left to right: Kelley Milloy, Laura (Kozon) Atkinson, Larissa Williams, Hillary (Lupo) Bufalino, Pia (Lenane) Cellamare, Amanda (Kratzer) Meyers, Katelin (Klepsch) Nelson

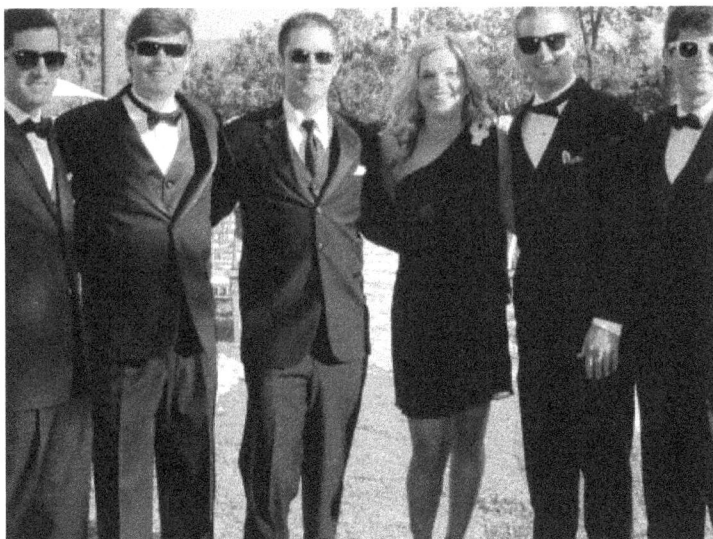

This picture was taken at my cousin's wedding in Pasadena, California in 2011. This was the first time my boyfriend, (at the time) Evan, met all of my boy cousins and extended family!
From left to right: Danny, Byron, Evan, me, Ben, and Sam. Apparently they forgot to tell me I needed sunglasses to be in the picture!

This is the very first half marathon I ever did. It was the Go! St. Louis race. I fell in love with running that day and have continued to do races every year since then. To date, I've completed eight half marathons!

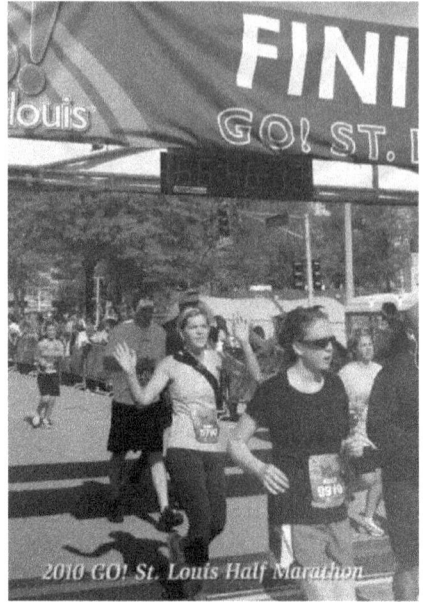

2010 GO! St. Louis Half Marathon

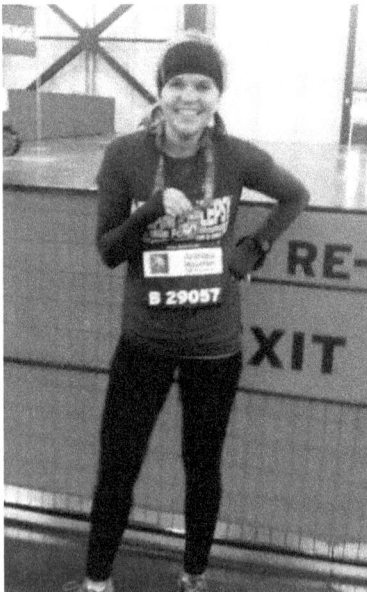

This was the first half marathon I did where I raised money to run. I was on Team Epilepsy in Houston and raised nearly $1,000 for the Epilepsy Foundation of Texas. It was also the race where I PR'd. That personal record still stands today!

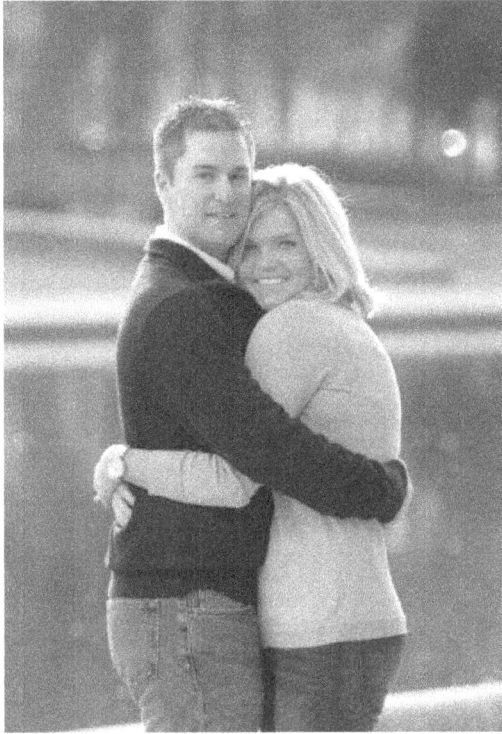

My Ev.
Here we are in 2012
after getting engaged
in Houston.

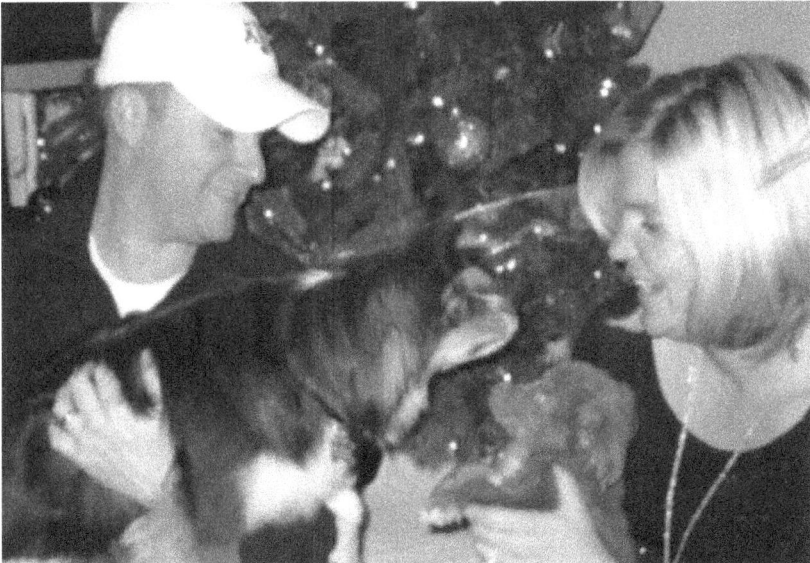

Evan and I are happiest spending time with our two loves,
Huey Lewis and Teddy Bear. This was Teddy's first
Christmas… December 2014. Teddy was only 12 weeks old.

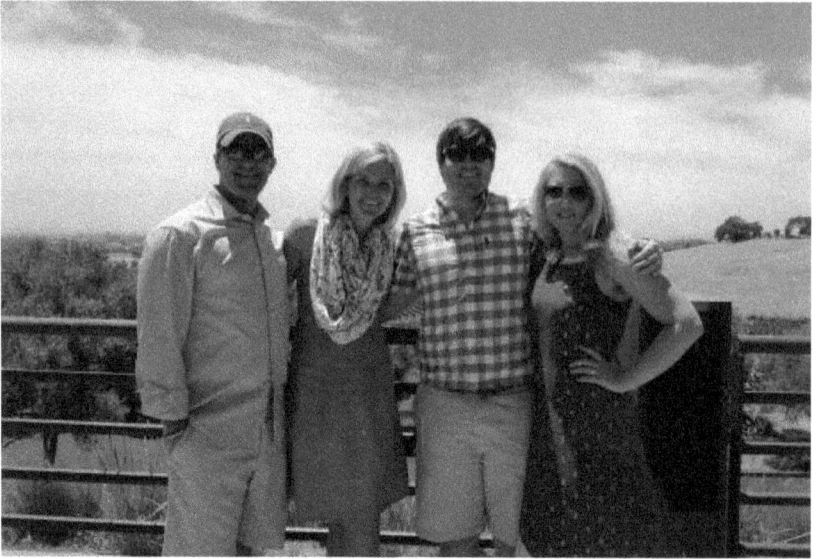

In Napa with Evan, Byron, and Byron's now wife, Allison. We all went to Napa to celebrate Byron and Allison's engagement. Evan and I fell in love with Napa and can't wait to go back!

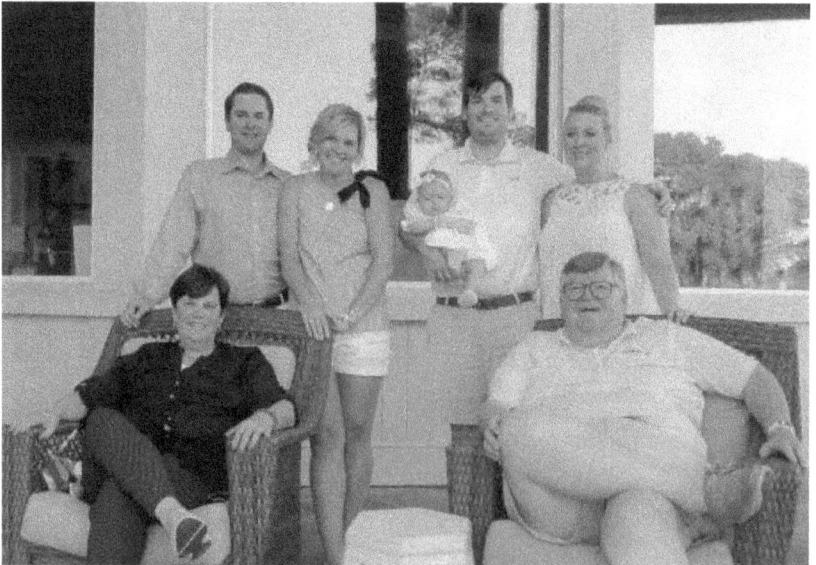

The Gustus family is expanding. This is our most recent family photo from this year's family vacation to Hilton Head Island. In the back you have Evan and me, my brother, Byron, and his wife, Allison, and our whole family's new, little bundle of joy, Caroline.

LOOKING BACK

My time as a young adult living at Purdue and then on my own with epilepsy in Chicago and St. Louis was interesting to say the least. I was independent but still a little dependent. I was self-sufficient but still needed some help. I was on my own, but always had a strong support system of family and friends.

At every major intersection of my life, I've always been blessed with at least one special person who I knew would always be there for me. Those are the people that have shaped who I am today. I am confident in my skin, and most people would never know that I'm epileptic. That's because it never mattered to my family or any of my close friends. Therefore, it never mattered to me (well, for the most part). I had health problems, but they still wanted me to live a happy, healthy, independent life. And, guess what? Because of them, I can say with confidence I did and I still am!

I feel very lucky that at every major cross-roads in my life, I had a new person (I consider all of them angels) waiting for me... to be that support system. To be that friend. To be that caregiver when I needed it most.

In college, I had Kelley.

In New York City, I had Laura.

In grad school, I had Jackie.

Once I moved back to St. Louis for my first real job, I had Leia.

To all of them, I am eternally thankful. While I was writing this book, I'll never forget it... I texted Kelley, "BTW, reliving all of this... I never said thank you to you for being such a good friend...

157

You never once made me feel bad or anything about having epilepsy. Love you so much!!!"

Her response, "Oh my gosh, yes you have! You've said thank you lots. I swear. And you *never* should have to. You'd do the same for me."

She is right. I would do the exact same for Kelley. And I'd do the same for Laura, Jackie, and Leia.

TEN

A Note to a Younger Me

"Not all of us can do great things, but we can do small things with great love."

MOTHER TERESA

There are a couple things that I wish I could sit my 14 year old self down and say, so I'm going to do that for you now.

ALWAYS TAKE YOUR MEDICINE

Just because you think you don't need it and feel frustrated that nobody else around you has to take medicine as religiously as you do, put your big girl or big boy pants on and deal with it! Just take it. Take it on time. Every time. I think some of my seizures could have been prevented if I had just gotten over the fact that I didn't like medicine sooner.

YOU ARE DIFFERENT AND THAT'S OKAY

Don't be mad about it! Learn from it. Grow from it. In high school, when you are getting TP'd from missing the soccer sleepover and benched because you're moving a little slower than you used to, it's hard to see past that. And believe me, everybody would agree you have the right to be mad.

Refocus your anger and grow from those experiences. Turn it into something positive. Okay, so you can't play competitive sports anymore? Let's talk about all the amazing things you *can* do. I promise, there will be more than you'd ever imagine.

LISTEN TO YOUR BODY

Please. When your body is telling you it's too tired, just go home. Get some rest. There is always going to be another party. Missing one party when you are exhausted is not the end of the world, and it will most likely help you to not have a seizure. Your body will start to give you clues when you are starting to get overtired. Personally, I start to get auras. Some people in the medical community consider auras a form of a seizure. I do not. My auras consist of me feeling really bad de ja vu. It's a feeling that something is just not right. It's hard to explain, and if you don't have epilepsy, well, sorry. You are not in the cool kids club on this one, because unless you have it, you cannot really describe it.

Anyway, as time has passed, slowly auras have been classified as seizures. Well, I wholeheartedly disagree with that, but I will say that is a way for your body to offer a gentle nudge that you need to get some sleep. So, listen to it.

THE SEIZURES YOU HAVE NOW WILL INEVITABLY AFFECT YOU LATER

You may not know it now, but with every seizure you have, it's going to make it harder on your one and only brain. Seizures can cause memory problems. Seizures can cause word finding problems. Just know that when you think the only thing happening when you have a seizure is that you have to sit out for a day or two, it's just not true. There are long-term difficulties that you need to be prepared for.

I have had to come up with ways in my adult-life to accommodate my memory loss and word finding problems. It's extremely frustrating. At work, I keep a list of absolutely everything. I keep a notebook and every single thing we talk about in meetings and action items that come out of it, I write down. If you do not have seizures, you may be thinking, yeah, duh, that's a to-do list, I have one too. But, this is a to-do list on steroids. It's different.

For me, I start my day with a to-do list. Each item I do, I have to cross off with a different color pen. I have to keep record of every task on there and whether or not it has been completed, because sometimes I forget that I've done it. My notebook is my savior at work. I document meetings and what happens, because inevitably, next week when somebody asks a question about what happened, the information will be gone.

I also have word finding problems. If I had to talk about my biggest insecurity when it comes to seizures, word finding problems wins. I have been in meetings with entire leadership teams and clients and had the floor. I'll be talking in important situations and not be able to think of a critical word. That, for me, is embarrassing. I do not try to work around it, though. I stop and ask for help. I will say, "What is the word for...?" Then, I go on to describe the word I am trying to locate in my brain. The people I work with are very supportive and understanding and always help me figure it out.

I wish when I was in high school and college, somebody would have sat me down and helped me understand the long-term effects of seizures. I feel like nobody ever gave us information about future memory loss and word finding problems, and I often wonder if I knew that, would I have changed my behaviors sooner? I'd like to think, yes.

EVERYBODY CAN HANDLE THE TRUTH

Don't be afraid to tell people you have epilepsy. It's not worth it. Epilepsy is a part of who you are. It does not define you. It does not change who you are, but it's a part of you. People are not going to look at you and not want to be around you because you have epilepsy. People are going to want to know how to help you should something happen. I'm not saying that you have to introduce yourself, "Hi, I'm Abby. I'm Abby with epilepsy." No, I'm not saying that at all. I'm saying as the conversation allows, let the person or people you are around know. The more comfortable you are with the situation, the more comfortable those around you will be, and then, it's a non-issue. Give people the opportunity to accept it and ask questions before something major happens and chaos ensues.

FIND A WAY TO SAY "IT" THAT WORKS FOR YOU

First, don't be afraid to say, "I have epilepsy," but also find a way that works for you. For me, I often weave the fact that I have epilepsy into conversations about my volunteer activities. It just so happens that I like giving back to others and am an active volunteer in different Houston charities because so many people helped me along the way. Often when I talk about those activities, I can explain the "why" behind spending much of my extra time volunteering.

In fact, I've even worked it in at job interviews at this point. While I wasn't always comfortable telling my employers about epilepsy, eventually I got to a point where I felt it was only fair to tell them. (*IMPORTANT DISCLAIMER:* You are in no way obligated to tell potential employers about your seizures if you do not want to. I made a choice to tell them.) I wanted my potential employers to know that when I do have a seizure, it typically takes me 24 to 48 hours to fully recover.

I've only worked for two companies in my career, but when I left McCarthy to come to CBRE in the summer of 2013, I made the decision to tell my now boss about my seizures. I happened to be interviewing with two people at a Starbucks.

"So, Abby, tell us something that you are most proud of in your career or personal life, whatever you are most proud of," Kristi, my boss now said to me.

"Well, for me, it's living a happy and successful life with epilepsy," I said. Most people find it impressive when you overcome an obstacle. I got that off my chest the very first day I met my boss, and she has been more than supportive every day since then.

KNOWLEDGE IS POWER

My parents taught me this. I would always get frustrated at my mom when we would go to doctor's appointments. My whole goal was to get an updated prescription and get the heck out of there. My mom used those opportunities to ask about new treatments available. Are there any new drugs on the market? What are other people doing to treat epilepsy? Are those treatments working? Are there any studies going on right now? Have there been any interesting new research findings released?

While I never cared, my parents did… a lot. I wish I would have cared more. The sooner you take ownership of your health and your treatments, the better off you will be. My mom was not willing to "settle" with the side effects of the first few drugs we tried. I wish I wouldn't have been either. The knowledge we gained by her (annoying at the time) questions changed my future and my fate with epilepsy.

FIND THE RIGHT BALANCE FOR YOU

No doubt about it, the "balance" that I have to have in my life is significantly different than my peers. This can include anything and everything from going out with friends for a drink after work or needing to work extra hours when a big project is due or even training for a half marathon. My "balance" looks very different from that of my peers who don't live their day to day lives with epilepsy. I have to plan for those types of events to ensure I don't get overtired… to ensure my stress levels stay somewhat stable… to ensure that my body is not overworked. There are many times where a bad decision to stay out late with friends has ended up with me having a seizure. Over time, I've learned those limits. I surround myself with people who understand and appreciate those limits and support my health.

Finding a balance takes time. But, start to recognize those triggers and slowly change your habits for the better.

SURROUND YOURSELF WITH SUPPORTIVE PEOPLE

These are people who understand what it means when you say, "I need to go to bed, I'm tired." They do not try to convince you otherwise.

These are people who understand what it means at work when you say, "I've hit my limit." They ask how they can help and what you need to make the project or task at hand work.

Find those people. The people who say okay and support whatever it is you need to do to put your health first are the people to seek out and surround yourself with.

ELEVEN

Right Where I Need to Be

"Where there is love there is life."

MAHATMA GANDHI

After a few years in St. Louis, I was getting antsy. I loved it there, but I knew that I did not want to live there my whole life, for whatever reason. Getting away to Purdue, Chicago, and New York City gave me the feeling that this was not ever going to be my forever home.

I was loving life, I had one of my best friends literally one street over, but for some reason, I knew I didn't want to live in St. Louis anymore. Not because I didn't love the city, not because I wasn't enjoying it, something was just tugging at me to move to a bigger city with more "action."

As luck would have it, these feelings of needing something more came right around that time that McCarthy was looking to open a Houston office. They were going to need a marketing person for that office. I happened to know the person who they were planning to appoint to lead the office in Houston and lobbied for the job.

I had never been to Houston in my entire life. I did not know anything about it, but I wanted to go. I wanted to be in Texas and really didn't know why. In the Fall of 2010, I was offered the Marketing Coordinator position in Houston and took it. Note to self, when you re-locate for a company, there should be some incentive attached to it. Just because you want to move there does not mean you should not be compensated for it. Just a small tidbit for anybody who wanted it!

My mom and I went to visit one time to pick out an apartment, just like we did in Chicago. I was thinking, god, I hope I like this place! At least I had visited Chicago before committing to move there. What was I thinking?!

McCarthy did already have people in the city that I knew as acquaintances, so they were able to give me some recommendations of where to look for a place. Once again, I felt like Dorothy from the Wizard of Oz… we're not in St. Louis anymore, Abby. Rent prices are much higher. So, I was back to a one bedroom, with a little nook for an office in Midtown, just outside downtown Houston. It was actually a really nice place. I literally could see Houston's beautiful skyline from my apartment balcony. I spent a lot of time out there, because I loved the view so much.

My mom helped me move the first weekend of December in 2010. I remember it very well. The plan was that we would drive down in my car and meet the moving truck at the new apartment. She would stay the weekend to help me unpack and fly back to St. Louis on Sunday night.

That was by far the longest I had ever spent in a car in my entire life. That drive felt like it was never going to end! Since then, I've already driven back and forth a couple times, but I just remember thinking that very first time, when will we be there?!

We unpacked almost everything and had boxes piling up. Some of the McCarthy guys that I knew as acquaintances called to "check in" on me and see if we needed any help. Turned out, by Saturday afternoon, we did need help.

"Actually, I could use a couple guys over here to haul all of the moving boxes to the trash, if you don't mind," I said when they called.

Within 30 minutes, a group of construction guys were at my apartment to save the day and help us de-clutter the already cramped space! It was a Saturday, and as the group of guys were leaving, one of the said, "Hey Abby, we're going to a bar down the street in an hour or so, you should come have a drink."

I looked at my mom, "Yeah, that sounds fun! I'll text you!"

After they left, I turned to my mom, "I actually do want to go out. One of my friends from Purdue lives here, and I would like to go meet him out. Are you going to be okay here by yourself?"

"Yes. I'm going to lie down and turn on Lifetime," she said to me.

"That actually sounds really nice to me, but I'd like to go out if you don't mind," I responded. As soon as my mom said that, though, I knew she'd be just fine. That's what we both do when we are exhausted and just want to veg out.

I hopped in the shower and was ready for my first night out in Houston!

OH, WHAT A NIGHT

This was only my second time ever in my life in this city, and I was headed out for a night on the town! I had one friend from Purdue in Houston, who actually happened to be from St. Louis too, so we hit it off. I called him, and we decided to meet at a bar called Pub Fiction, just down the street from my new apartment.

I asked my mom to drop me off at the bar (even though I could have walked) since I did not know where I was going. Cool move, Abby. We didn't have Uber back then, okay?!

Either way, she dropped me off and I hopped out.

"Hey, Abs, you told those guys from work you would text them today when they helped us. You really should do that."

"Yeah. Okay," I actually had absolutely no intentions of texting them, but she was right. They helped us a lot that day. So, I listened and texted them.

They must have been next door or close by, because in walked a group of about six guys about 20 minutes later. I knew all of them, but stuck near my friend Allen from Purdue, because that's who I knew well and was comfortable with.

I slowly became more relaxed and started talking to all of the McCarthy guys that showed up. They were all really nice guys. I was excited to have the opportunity to work with them.

The scene at Pub Fiction got a little boring, so we all decided to move the party to the next bar called Howl at the Moon. We walked in, and before I knew it, a guy named Evan put his arm around me, pulled me to the bar, and said, "Welcome to Texas! Let me buy you a shot of Tequila!"

I thought he was super cute, so I said, okay. I smiled and he ordered two shots and two beers. I was instantly taken by Evan. What makes me laugh now, looking back on it all, is that on my one visit down to Texas, McCarthy wanted me to tour the job-site where we had a team working. Evan happened to be the job-site tour guide a month or two prior to this night, and it was the most boring job-site tour of a McCarthy job-site I'd ever taken in my life!

I couldn't believe this was the same guy!

It was one of those absolutely fun and crazy nights. Once again, yes, I have seizures. And yes, I did drink alcohol. Not excessively, but socially. You learn your limits.

Evan walked me home, thank goodness, and we kissed goodnight.

That, in turn, meant I wanted to hide my face forever and never see him again! How did I let this happen?!?! I worked for three years at the headquarters of McCarthy in St. Louis and never went on one date with any of the guys I worked with.

I'm in Houston for a new job and within 48 hours, I kissed one of the guys I had to work with! What was wrong with me?!? And, on top of everything, my mom was at my apartment! This was bad. This was very, very bad.

I was so mad at myself when I woke up. I knew a) my mom had seen me feeling no pain which was embarrassing enough, b) that I kissed a guy I was going to have to see again... at work nonetheless, and c) that I was about to be late for brunch with my mom, my new boss, and his wife!

I showered quickly as my mom asked me question and question about the night before. Every five seconds, my phone would buzz.

New text message.

"Who is that?!?"

"UMMMMM… it's Evan."

"So, who's Evan?"

"Tell him to leave me alone."

New text message.

New text message.

New text message.

"Oh. My. God. What is wrong with that guy?" I said to my mom.

My mom was laughing. Evan was sending *a lot* of text messages to me the day after we went out.

"I think he wants to see you again," my mom said laughing.

"Oh my god, well, I don't want to see him," I said, but I was lying. I wanted to see Evan again really bad. I could have gone without the excessive number of texts the next day, although they did make me laugh.

THE ONE

After that night, we were inseparable. Evan was my new city tour guide. He had a Jeep Wrangler at the time, so we would cruise around Houston with the top off. You can do that pretty much year round here, which is one of the many reasons I'm so attached to this city. You cannot beat the weather! It was December, and we were riding around in the Jeep in just jeans and a long sleeve shirt. I loved it.

He would try to teach me how to drive his stick shift Wrangler, but I ended up stalling out almost every time. Once, I stalled out in the middle of River Oaks Boulevard at the four way stop right in front of the Country Club. People were honking, and Evan was sitting next to me laughing!

"It's not funny Ev!!! HELP!"

Insert inaudible laughing from Evan here.

Finally, I was able to inch us through to the other side of the four way stop so we could switch seats.

It was really funny… *after* we got through the intersection. And still, to this day, I cannot drive a stick shift.

It was not long after our first night out that Evan took me on our first official date to Brenner's on the Bayou. It's still one of my favorite places to eat in the entire world, because it reminds me of our first date. The food is delicious too, but I love thinking about that night.

I loved Evan, and he loved me. He was the perfect fit for me. He knew about my seizures from the very beginning of our relationship. I never even wanted to hide it from him. As always, I'm convinced, everything happens for a reason. Evan's dad, my father-in-law, has epilepsy, too. Evan has never actually seen his dad have a seizure, but he understood enough about it when we met to feel compassion and empathy towards me and the fact that I was living with it. It also never scared him, which I think is a huge testament to Evan. He took it in stride and loved me for me, and that was all I ever wanted in my life partner.

TWELVE

Reflections

"Go forward in life with a twinkle in your eye and a smile on your face,
but with great purpose in heart."
GORDON B. HINCKLEY

My journey has led me here to the perfect place. I truly
believe that I am exactly where I am supposed to be in my life. Every
step of this journey, every heartache, every seizure, led me to where
I'm at now… happy and healthy. It's clear to me that each person
I've connected with has come into my life for a reason. There are
no coincidences. Everything happens for a reason. Things happen
to help us learn and grow. While my experiences are strongly tied
to epilepsy, powerful lessons come from any crisis, and that's what
I chose to focus on, the lessons that helped me grow as a person.

It's clear that my health has significantly improved from
when I was a teenager and young adult. That's because the initial
intensity of my anger and frustration with my diagnosis has
lessened. The resentment towards the fact that I was different from
my friends has tapered. The bitterness I had about taking eight pills
a day is gone. The days turned into months, months to years, and

now it's reality. The new reality is that life… with epilepsy… is forever. I'm okay with that too, because I have chosen a life of love, gratitude, and happiness.

In my journey, I've endured some serious setbacks. I still encounter setbacks today. But, that's okay. I'm thriving. Each new hurdle provides me the opportunity to show my strength again. Each new setback gives me the opportunity to learn and grow. And then, I can share that knowledge with the children I work with at the Epilepsy Foundation. That's what makes me happy. I find happiness in helping people, and I realized as I talked to more and more people, that just hearing my story gave them hope. Just hearing that I went through the same thing inspired them.

I always find myself looking back, reflecting on all the ups and downs we've had, thinking, how do I want this story to end? But, that's just it… it's not over. It's still going, and I want it to be positive. I want people to look at me and feel inspired, that they, too, can lead a fulfilling and successful life. I am grateful every morning for the chance to add another anecdote to this blessed story I'm able to tell. If my past is any sign of my future, there are many amazing chapters to come. One day at a time… one new adventure at a time… I'm still writing.

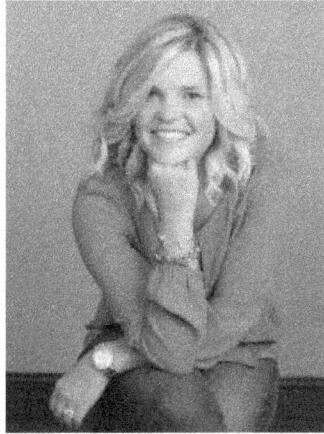

Author Abby Gustus Alford

At the age of 14, Abby Gustus Alford was diagnosed with epilepsy. After some tough years, she went on to graduate with two college degrees and her Master's in Journalism. She started working professionally in St. Louis then moved to Texas. Since moving to Houston, Abby has been very involved in epilepsy awareness and advocacy. She currently serves as a Transition Program mentor for the Epilepsy Foundation of Texas. In addition to her volunteer work with the Epilepsy Foundation, Abby has been quoted in the *Enlighten: Action for Epilepsy* 10th anniversary coffee table book and is a contributing blogger to the *Living Well with Epilepsy* website.

Abby's intimate, first-hand knowledge of the challenges that come with successfully coping with a diagnosis of epilepsy offers a unique perspective for both parents and teens. She has found through her volunteer work with the Epilepsy Foundation of Texas having someone to talk to about real life experiences, beyond the medical community, is necessary and helpful. Her network within the epilepsy community is continuously growing as she spreads her message of hope and works with people to assure them that they too can lead happy, healthy lives with epilepsy.

Seize the Day was written to encourage teens and adults to live the life they have always dreamed of, with an understanding of the emotional and physical struggles one with epilepsy and their families encounter.

Her success in her marketing career brought her to Texas, where she now works as the Training and Communications Manager for a global commercial real estate firm and lives a happy and healthy life with her husband, Evan, and their pride and joy puppies, Huey and Teddy.

www.ingramcontent.com/pod-product-compliance
Lightning Source LLC
Chambersburg PA
CBHW032352280326
41935CB00008B/542